Professionalism in Medicine

Professionalism in Medicine

JILL THISTLETHWAITE

General Practitioner
Medical Educator
Office of Postgraduate Medical Education
University of Sydney

and

JOHN SPENCER

General Practitioner
Medical Educator
Sub-Dean for Primary and Community Care
Newcastle University

Foreword by

SEAN HILTON

Professor of Primary Care and Deputy-Principal for Teaching and Learning
St George's, University of London

Radcliffe Publishing
Oxford • New York

Radcliffe Publishing Ltd
18 Marcham Road
Abingdon
Oxon OX14 1AA
United Kingdom

www.radcliffe-oxford.com
Electronic catalogue and worldwide online ordering facility.

British Library Cataloguing in Publication Data

A catalogue record for this book is available from the British Library.

ISBN-13: 978 185775 763 7

Typeset by Pindar New Zealand (Egan Reid), Auckland, New Zealand
Printed and bound by TJI Digital, Padstow, Cornwall, UK

Contents

Foreword   vii

About the authors   ix

1 The context   1

2 Learning from history   17

3 The code of conduct: professionalism, law and ethics   36

4 Professional–patient relationships   52

5 Communication and its relationship with professionalism   69

6 Cultural diversity and competence   89

7 Professional knowledge and development: keeping up to date   102

8 Personal development and self-care   117

9 The nature of autonomy for the professional and the patient   134

10 Learning and teaching professionalism   156

11 Assessing professionalism   185

12 Professionalism and social justice: the next step?   210

Index   223

I dedicate this book to George for his support and encouragement during its long gestation. JT

I dedicate this book to Jessie for her company in the wee small hours. JS

Foreword

Professionalism has come to the fore as a topic in medical education only in the last 20 years. Prior to that there was little reference to it in the literature, and yet – of course – it was there; tacit, implicit, accepted by patients and professionals alike. It is interesting to chart the emergence of this aspect of medicine, which now occupies such a prominent place in undergraduate and postgraduate medical curricula.

For centuries professions have held a particular niche in society. Original professions of medicine, law and the clergy arose in the early universities and guilds, but the notion of *profession* goes back at least as far as Hippocrates. Medicine is, in part, the modern embodiment of the ancient art of healing – present since the earliest days of civilisation. The role of the doctor has continued through centuries of societal development and change and has generally brought a (sometimes undeserved) high place in society's esteem. In modern times sociologists have attacked professions as self interested and protectionist rather than altruistic, but the reputation of the doctor has been maintained and enhanced by the great advances of medical science. Most recently, however, a backlash has occurred against medicine and the powerful culture of biomedicine. This backlash incorporates, amongst other features, societal changes towards consumerism; a 'blame culture' that, in turn, generates a 'risk management' culture, and politicisation of healthcare systems fuelled by public concerns and rising costs.

As healthcare delivery has become relentlessly more complex and – in the acute sector – more pressured and high technology, doctors' professionalism has come under challenge from all directions. Respected authors have written of the need to 'renegotiate' medicine's social contract, and official and regulatory bodies around the world have identified the need to re-emphasise the role of the doctor and the purposes of education and training. As medicine has had to redefine what it means by professionalism, medical education has had to dissect the components of this newly defined entity and consider how best to incorporate it into the curriculum and – a greater challenge – how to assess it in developmental and supportive ways.

And so, this book *Professionalism in Medicine* by Jill Thistlethwaite and John Spencer, is both welcome and timely. Both authors have long experience of medical education and of delivering medical care from the generalist perspective, and they have produced an admirable summary of the field. They have reviewed the history and context, and give an overview of the key literature. Chapters on the various aspects, or domains, of professionalism are presented in clear, comprehensively referenced format. Coverage is given to vital areas of ethical practice; communication; cultural sensitivity; and professional responsibilities including self-care. Chapters 10 and 11 address the challenges of curriculum development and assessment, and the final chapter tackles social responsibility for the profession – perhaps the most significant test of the adaptability of the profession. Unless our education and training instils the abilities and beliefs required to respond speedily to changing societal needs, the profession risks future marginalisation rather than leadership in delivery of healthcare.

Thistlethwaite and Spencer's book is an important addition to the field and will be of value to all those involved in medical and healthcare education, and to a wider audience interested in the development of those nascent professionals to whom we will be entrusting the future of medicine.

Professor Sean Hilton MD FRCGP
Deputy Principal
St George's, University of London
May 2008

About the authors

Associate Professor Jill Thistlethwaite is a medical educator and general practitioner. She trained in the UK and received her PhD in medical education from the University of Maastricht. From 1996 to 2003 she was senior lecturer in community-based education at Leeds University School of Medicine. In late 2003 she moved to Australia and was Associate Professor in General Practice and Rural Medicine at James Cook University in Townsville, North Queensland. Since 2006 she has been working at the Centre for Innovation in Professional Health Education and Research (CIPHER) at the University of Sydney. She works across undergraduate, postgraduate and continuing professional education. Dr Thistlethwaite chairs the Prevocational Education Sub-Committee of the Education Committee of the Royal Australian College of General Practitioners, is associate editor of the *Journal of Interprofessional Care* and is on the editorial advisory board of *Clinical Teacher*. She has published in a variety of education and clinical journals, and is co-author of two books published in 2006 – on consultation skills (for the Royal College of General Practitioners in the UK), and working with simulated patients.

Professor John Spencer is a general practitioner in Tyneside in North-East England, and Sub-Dean for Primary and Community Care at Newcastle University. He has 25 years' experience in health care education, predominantly undergraduate medical education, but also pre- and post-basic nurse training, vocational training for general practice, education and training for pharmacists and paramedics, continuing professional development and postgraduate training, dental and veterinary education, and staff development. He has published widely in the fields of both health services and educational research and development. Particular interests are teaching, learning and assessment of communication and professionalism, and user involvement in healthcare education. He is a Specialist Advisor to the Higher Education Academy Subject Centre for Medicine, Dentistry and Veterinary Medicine, has been actively involved with the Association for the Study of Medical Education for many years, and is deputy editor of *Medical Education* and Editor in Chief of *Clinical Teacher*.

CHAPTER 1

The context

This chapter explores:
- the historical context
- what's in a word – definitions of professionalism
- the origins of the recent interest in professionalism
- the UK experience
- developments in North America
- trust in doctors
- patient-centred professionalism.

> A professional is a man who can do his job when he doesn't feel like it.
> An amateur is a man who can't do his job when he does feel like it.[1]
>
> *James Agate (1877–1947), British diarist and critic*

HISTORICAL CONTEXT

Doctors have been considered 'professionals' for as long as the concept of a profession has existed. Since Hippocrates' time in Western cultures, and for at least as long in Oriental cultures (e.g. China), doctors have held a special place in their communities, operating through an implicit social contract. In return for deploying their special (and usually carefully guarded) knowledge and skills, and being seen to act in a principled manner in the best interests of their patients, the privilege of autonomy and the freedom to self-regulate was bestowed upon them, as well as considerable social status. This arrangement endured for millennia, essentially unquestioned until well into the twentieth century, notwithstanding periodic assaults and critical analyses by sociologists, anthropologists, politicians, academics and patient/consumer groups. Nonetheless, the potential for doctors to act in an unethical manner and abuse their powerful status, or to act incompetently and harm patients but get away with it, was well recognised by both satirists (the famous line in George Bernard Shaw's play *A Doctor's Dilemma*, 'All professions are a conspiracy against the laity',[2] comes to mind) and philosophers (e.g. Ivan Illich in his scathing attack on medicine and the medical profession for the 'expropriation of health' in the mid-1970s[3]). However, it has only really been in the last 10 years or so that professionalism has come under intense scrutiny and stimulated such wide-ranging and far-reaching debate. Some of the reasons why this is so are briefly explored in this chapter, but first . . . what's in a word?

WHAT'S IN A WORD?

As most authors on the subject observe, one of the problems bedevilling discussion about 'professionalism' is its definition. The word is full of nuance and, as with such words as 'love' or 'quality', perhaps each of us is clear what *we* understand by the term, but we find it difficult to articulate. In fact definitions of professionalism abound, and some of the more important ones that have emerged recently are discussed in this chapter (Hilton and Slotnik of St George's Medical School, London, suggested the most pithy to date, namely 'A reflective practitioner who acts ethically'[4]). However, if only to marvel at the richness of language, it is worth considering how the concepts of 'profession' and 'professional' may be understood by the general public. Many people would see a 'professional' as being the opposite of an 'amateur' – for example, in music or sport, in which context the professional is usually thought to have skills superior to those of the amateur, and is of course paid to perform or to compete. However, there was also the notion of the 'gentleman amateur' – the sportsman who did not sully himself by being paid to perform, unlike the professional who took money and thus demeaned the spirit of sportsmanship. A soldier or a killer may also be described as 'professional', which here implies carrying out a job with calculated efficiency without fuss or emotion. Interestingly, the word 'clinical' is sometimes also used in this context. Finally, a footballer or rugby player will be cautioned for committing a 'professional foul', a 'deliberate act of foul play, usually to prevent an opponent scoring.'[5]

WHY THE RECENT INTEREST IN MEDICAL PROFESSIONALISM?

Recent interest in medical professionalism, at least in the UK, dates back to the early 1990s. It could be argued that reform in undergraduate medical education, led as it was by the General Medical Council through its 1993 recommendations, *Tomorrow's Doctors*,[6] helped to catalyse thinking in this area. Although the word 'professionalism' was not used in the document, the principles were implicit – for example, with increased emphasis on communication skills, ethical reasoning, the development of appropriate attitudes, and so on. The recommendations and the visits that followed empowered educators in medical schools, previously marginalised, to develop teaching, learning and assessment in relevant areas, and raised awareness about the need to address these issues effectively and systematically.

In 1994, Sir Kenneth Calman, then Chief Medical Officer, published a paper in the *British Medical Journal* in which he argued that it was timely to consider the nature of professionalism, in the light of 'increasing public and professional interest in medicine, and a questioning of professional standards and the quality of care.'[7] He acknowledged that it was not easy to define 'a profession', but suggested that it was likely to have all or most of the characteristics listed in Box 1.1.

BOX 1.1 CHARACTERISTICS OF A PROFESSION[7]

- Driven by a sense of vocation or calling, implying service to others.
- Has a distinctive knowledge base, which is kept up to date.
- Sets its own standards and controls access through examination.
- Has a special relationship with those whom it serves.
- Is guided by particular ethical principles.
- Is self-regulating and accountable.

Calman offered a statement about what kind of doctors society needs and the requisite underlying attitudes and competencies. In essence he argued that 'Doctors need to have a broad vision of the world and be able to change and adapt as the knowledge base changes. They need to have outside interests and be rounded people, with breadth as well as depth.'[7] For Calman, the most important implication of all this was for medical education and training.

Later the same year, the British Medical Association (BMA) organised a 'summit meeting' of the profession's leaders to debate medicine's 'core values', and this was apparently the first such meeting for over 30 years.[8] The need to revisit these values was presented in a no-nonsense fashion by Sir Maurice Shock, former Rector of Lincoln College, Oxford, who argued that the profession had failed thus far to appreciate the massive shift in societal attitudes which had occurred, particularly the advent of the 'consumer society', in the context of unprecedented medical advances and changing demography. He contended that 'the doctor is different, the patient is different, and the medicine is different' – indeed, 'everything is different, except the way you organise yourselves.'[8]

The assembled great and good discussed six core values, namely confidence, confidentiality, competence, contract, community responsibility and commitment. One issue that taxed the participants was whether the doctor's responsibility began and ended with the patient in the consulting room (the traditional view), or whether it extended to other patients, the community and the healthcare system, and beyond (a broader and more political view). After much debate, the list of core values was enhanced thus:

➤ commitment
➤ integrity
➤ confidentiality
➤ caring
➤ competence
➤ responsibility
➤ compassion
➤ spirit of enquiry
➤ advocacy.

A report of the summit meeting was duly published.[9]

Around the same time, the General Medical Council (GMC) was discussing proposals to shift the focus of its guidance to doctors away from a list of things that they must *not* do (the historic position, laid out in what was known as the 'Blue Book'), to a description of what a good doctor *should* do. These guidelines were published as *Duties of a Doctor*[10] and *Good Medical Practice*.[11] In *Good Medical Practice* (GMP), the GMC outlined 'the principles and values on which good practice is founded', and although the guidance was predominantly addressed to the profession, it was also intended to inform the public about what they should and could expect from their doctors. This signified a major change in the focus of thinking about the purpose of such guidance, although interestingly the actual word 'professionalism' was not used in the first edition.

The seven headings of *Good Medical Practice* will be familiar to most UK readers, having been adopted as the framework, among other things, for revalidation and appraisal, and the curriculum for the Foundation Programme for newly qualified doctors. The headings are shown in Box 1.2.

BOX 1.2 THE SEVEN HEADINGS OF *GOOD MEDICAL PRACTICE* [11]

- Good clinical care
- Maintaining good medical practice
- Teaching and training, appraising and assessment
- Relationships with patients
- Working with colleagues
- Probity
- Health

The 'bottom line' of *Good Medical Practice* was that patients must be able to trust doctors with their lives and health, and that doctors should make the care of their patients their first priority.

Although Calman's paper, the BMA report and *Good Medical Practice* doubtless promoted debate and discussion, it is arguable that they had little impact on the 'doctor on the Clapham omnibus.' Sadly, that required the stimulus of external forces. The Bristol paediatric heart surgery scandal, news of which broke in early 1996 through the satirical magazine *Private Eye*, could be said to be the point at which the public and the Government *really* began to take an interest in professionalism. Other cases followed Bristol – for example, that of Rodney Ledward and Richard Neale, two wayward gynaecologists who were eventually struck off the GMC register on grounds of serious professional misconduct, and of course the mass-murdering GP Harold Fred Shipman.

The 1998 Bristol Inquiry, chaired by Professor Ian Kennedy, identified a catalogue of lapses in professionalism at both individual and team levels, and also serious failure within the organisation. The Inquiry's report (known as the Kennedy Report) was a no-holds-barred indictment of an anachronistic mode of professionalism, characterised by paternalism, misplaced collegiality (described as a 'club culture'), failure of self-regulation and ultimately failure to protect patients.[12] This had come about precisely as Maurice Shock had said, because changes in medical culture had not kept pace with changing societal values and expectations. In the words of Sir Donald Irvine, President of the GMC at the time, Bristol 'signalled the moment at which change became inevitable.'[13] Richard Smith, then editor of the *British Medical Journal*, was even more forthright. Quoting Yeats, 'All changed, changed utterly', he suggested the implications were so profound that Bristol would prove more important to the future of healthcare in the UK than any number of Government White Papers, and that its ramifications would be felt for years to come.[14] The list of issues raised by the Bristol Inquiry was long and challenging, largely focused around the need for greater accountability and improved self-regulation.[10] Inevitably the role of the GMC was heavily criticised, and the report catalysed major change in both its organisation and function, which at the time of writing are still continuing. Smith (and others) exhorted the profession to 'maintain the impetus for improvement . . . and turn the fine words into effective action.'[14]

NORTH AMERICAN DEVELOPMENTS

It was not only in the UK that such deliberations were taking place. For example, the American Board of Internal Medicine (ABIM) established the Professionalism Project in 1992. The aims of the latter were to define professionalism and raise awareness in all those within internal medicine, and to provide a means for including professionalism within training curricula. Recommendations were published in 1994,[15] including the requirement that doctors seeking board certification, and hence medical registration, should *demonstrate* that they have acquired the values of professionalism. A transatlantic collaboration between the American College of Physicians and the American Society of Internal Medicine, the ABIM and the European Federation of Internal Medicine, known as the Medical Professionalism Project, followed this in 1999. The aim was to produce guidance for the new millennium, to which all medical professionals could and should aspire. The Project approached the problem from a different starting point, the basic premise being that medicine's commitment to the patient was being challenged by a wide range of factors. These included the technological and information revolution, changes in demography and healthcare delivery, the twin threats of bioterrorism and globalisation, and changing market forces. As a consequence, doctors were finding it increasingly difficult to fulfil their responsibilities to their patients. In this respect, the debate in the USA was more explicitly a response to what one author described as 'the corporate transformation' or 'industrialisation' of healthcare[16] than it was to scandals such as Bristol and Shipman, as in the UK.

Whatever the case, the new millennium provided an opportunity to reaffirm the basic principles of professionalism in a way that might help to reform healthcare. The product was a 'charter', which was published simultaneously in 2002 on both sides of the Atlantic in the *Lancet* and the *Annals of Internal Medicine*.[17] The basic tenets were familiar. The foundation of medicine's contract with society is 'professionalism', the elements of which must be clearly understood by both the profession and society. Underpinning this contract is public trust in doctors, which depends upon their integrity. The charter consisted of three fundamental principles and a set of professional responsibilities (*see* Box 1.3).

BOX 1.3 MEDICAL PROFESSIONALISM IN THE NEW
MILLENNIUM: A PHYSICIAN CHARTER[17]

Medical professionalism is underpinned by:

Three fundamental principles
- Primacy of patient welfare
- Primacy of patient autonomy
- Principle of social justice

Ten professional responsibilities
- Professional competence
- Honesty with patients
- Patient confidentiality
- Maintaining appropriate relationships with patients
- Improving quality of care
- Improving access to care
- Just distribution of resources
- Scientific knowledge
- Maintaining trust by managing conflicts of interest
- Professional responsibilities

The principles were uncompromisingly political. The primacy of patient welfare is based on altruism, which must not be compromised by factors such as market forces or political and administrative demands. Respect for patient autonomy involves doctors empowering patients to make informed decisions about their treatment, but this has to take place within an ethical framework. Finally, doctors must strive to promote social justice – for example, through fairer distribution of resources and by challenging discriminatory policies and practices. These principles were developed further in the set of responsibilities, which highlighted both individual and broader professional obligations. Whilst acknowledging that the practice of medicine was embedded in diverse cultures and value systems, and subject to different and wide-ranging pressures, the authors of the charter intended it 'to promote an action agenda . . . universal in scope and purpose.'[17]

In the context of the threats to professionalism described above, Herbert M Swick (of the Institute of Medicine and Humanities, Montana) proposed a 'normative definition' – one that was grounded in the everyday work of physicians, and their interactions with patients and families, and with their colleagues.[16] He intended it to be 'precise and inclusive' so as to have relevance for a wide constituency within the medical profession. He proposed a set of nine behaviours (*see* Box 1.4). As a professional, a physician must:

➤ subordinate their own interests to those of others (including managing conflicts of interest such that patient needs remain paramount)

➤ adhere to high ethical and moral standards (if their work has a high moral and social value, it follows that doctors must behave morally – 'Patients have a right to expect no less')

➤ respond to the needs of society (reflecting the 'compact' between the profession and the communities they serve)

➤ display core humanistic values (including integrity and trustworthiness, compassion and altruism – 'The practice of medicine is a human endeavour')

➤ exercise both individual and collective accountability (in return for the bestowed privilege of autonomy)

➤ demonstrate a continuing commitment to excellence (whilst recognising their limitations) as well as to scholarship and advancement

➤ deal with a high level of complexity and uncertainty (characterised by exercising independent judgement)

➤ reflect upon their actions and decisions (ultimately to bring balance to professional and personal life).

BOX 1.4 SWICK'S 'NORMATIVE' DEFINITION OF PROFESSIONALISM[16]

Medical professionalism comprises the following set of behaviours:
- Physicians subordinate their own interests to the interests of others.
- Physicians adhere to high ethical and moral standards.
- Physicians respond to societal needs.
- Physicians evince core humanistic values.
- Physicians exercise accountability for themselves and for their colleagues.
- Physicians demonstrate a commitment to excellence.
- Physicians exhibit a commitment to scholarship and to advancing their field.
- Physicians deal with high levels of complexity and uncertainty.
- Physicians reflect upon their actions and decisions.

As a response to the 'industrialisation' of medicine, Swick felt that it was important to reiterate aspects of professionalism that pertained to its social functions, not least because 'Without a strong sense of the public and social purposes served by professional knowledge, professionals tend to lose their distinctive voice in public debate.'[16]

Meanwhile, in Canada, the Royal College of Physicians and Surgeons had initiated a project, known as CanMEDS2000, to reform postgraduate education and ensure that all programmes were responsive to societal needs. The result was a framework describing a set of 'competencies' clustered into seven main roles.[18] The role of 'medical expert' lay at the heart of the CanMEDS framework, the others being 'manager', 'communicator', 'scholar', 'collaborator', 'health advocate' and 'professional.' The underlying principles of the last were that physicians should deliver highest-quality care with integrity, honesty and compassion, and should be committed to the health and well-being of individuals and society through ethical practice, professionally led regulation, and high personal standards of behaviour. A list of 14 'enabling competencies' expanded the basic principle. The framework was carefully implemented and has now been incorporated into accreditation, assessment and standards at all levels of medical education.

PROFESSIONALISM MUST BE TAUGHT

In parallel with the emerging literature that was attempting to 'nail down' the complexities of professionalism and its place in the modern world, educators were also starting to discuss and debate the challenges of teaching about professionalism. That it *must* be taught was not in question – the challenge was how and when, and in particular how it might be reliably assessed. Sylvia and Richard Cruess from Montreal offered some fundamental principles to guide educators.[19] They suggested that there should be identifiable content in undergraduate medical curricula, reinforced in postgraduate programmes and continuing professional development. Important concepts to highlight include altruism and the notion of 'calling', knowledge of codes of ethics, understanding the nature and limitations of individual and collective autonomy, and making explicit the links between professional status and societal obligations. Relevant material should be drawn from a wide range of disciplines outside medicine, including sociology, moral philosophy, economics and political science, so as to avoid allowing the profession 'to build and maintain its own myths while avoiding ideas challenging them.'[19] Other authors discussed ways of increasing students' self-awareness as a way of promoting better patient care,[20] or helping them to develop a sense of social responsibility through learning and working in the community.[21] Quoting Kenneth Berns, they contended that 'essentially the goal of medical education must now be to turn out Renaissance physicians – individuals capable of addressing patients' needs from the level of their molecules to the level of their participation in society.'[20] Another helpful contribution to thinking on the subject came from Hilton and Slotnick, who proposed a developmental model which saw professionalism not as a trait, but as an acquired state.[4] They defined six domains of professionalism (ethical practice, reflection and self-awareness, responsibility for action, respect for patients, teamwork, and social responsibility) which, they argued, are developed through experience, and reflection on experience, in parallel with the development of technical competence. They defined the early phase of this as 'proto-professionalism', and discussed some of the factors that both enable and hinder the process.

Thus as the new millennium dawned, 'medical professionalism' was high on the agenda of a wide range of stakeholders, including politicians, regulators, academics, educators, practitioners and, not least, the general public. A steady stream of publications about professionalism, what it is and how to teach and assess it, flowed from the major journals. Medical education conferences dedicated symposia and workshops to the topic. Regulatory bodies, such as the GMC, and policy makers wrestled with the issues.

A QUESTION OF TRUST

In 2002, Onora O'Neill, philosopher and ethicist, and Principal of Newnham College at Cambridge, gave the BBC Reith Lectures on the subject of 'trust'.[22] Her thought-provoking central thesis was that, despite received wisdom and extensive media hyperbole, the evidence in support of a supposed 'crisis in trust' was mixed. She argued that failures and abuse of trust were by no means new phenomena, and that despite the rhetoric, the evidence of increased *un*trustworthiness was thin. Actions speak louder than words, and if anything it seemed that people were placing as much trust in professionals and institutions as they had ever done before, albeit perhaps in a climate of increasing suspicion. This was perversely creating new situations which were worsening the problem. She singled out the human rights movement, new approaches to accountability, the media's apparent mission to spread suspicion and undermine trust, and new ideals of transparency. 'Rights' were promulgated without consideration of reciprocal responsibilities and obligations. The new bureaucratic accountability – including audit, league tables and performance targets – was distorting the proper aims of professional performance rather than enhancing it, and was damaging professional morale and integrity. She called for an 'intelligent' accountability that, among other things, would involve less top-down micro-management and a greater margin of responsible self-government. She used the recommendations of the Kennedy Report as an example of this kind of approach.[12] The pursuit of truth and transparency, she felt, was also paradoxically damaging and unhelpful: 'Increasing transparency can produce a flood of unsorted information and mis-information that provides little but confusion unless it can be sorted and assessed. It may add to uncertainty rather than to trust.'[22] She considered that a more effective strategy would be to reduce deception rather than to increase transparency. She suggested that claims about a crisis of trust were evidence of an unrealistic hankering after a world of total safety and compliance in which breaches of trust were totally eliminated, and that some of the 'new' institutions might actually be more damaging to trust than nurturing it: 'Plants don't flourish when we pull them up too often to check how their roots are growing; political, institutional and professional life too may not flourish if we constantly uproot it to demonstrate that everything is transparent and trustworthy.' To avoid a 'crisis of trustworthiness' brought about by the use of measures designed to stem the *supposed* crisis in trust, she concluded, we need to start communicating more openly.[22]

In 2004, the King's Fund published the results of a consultation exercise exploring medical professionalism.[23] Its main aim was to promote further debate, but also to offer a way forward, at least on some issues. They called for renewed emphasis on ensuring that patients' interests were at the heart of professional practice. They suggested the need for a new and explicit compact between government, the profession and the public in tune with prevailing values and expectations, strengthening medical leadership, and clarifying the relationship between doctors and managers. The same year the Royal College of Physicians established a Working Party to define the nature and role of medical professionalism in modern society. After an extensive inquiry, involving a literature review, oral and written evidence from a wide range of witnesses and informants sampling both medical and lay opinion, and questionnaire surveys and focus groups, it published its report in December 2005.[24] The basic principles of medical professionalism were revisited, and although it covered familiar territory, it took thinking about professionalism a few bold strides forward, not least in putting professionalism firmly in the context of partnership with patients. The report defined professionalism as 'a set of values, behaviours and relationships that underpins the trust that the public has in doctors', and further elaborated this in a description of medical professionalism (*see* Box 1.5).

BOX 1.5 ROYAL COLLEGE OF PHYSICIANS' DESCRIPTION
OF MEDICAL PROFESSIONALISM[24]

Medicine is a vocation in which a doctor's knowledge, clinical skills and judgement are put in the service of protecting and restoring human well-being. This purpose is realised through a partnership between patient and doctor, one based on mutual respect, individual responsibility and appropriate accountability.

In their day-to-day practice, doctors are committed to:
- integrity
- compassion
- altruism
- continuous improvement
- excellence
- working in partnership with members of the wider healthcare team.

These values, which underpin the science and practice of medicine, form the basis for a mutual contract between the medical profession and society. Each party has a duty to work to strengthen the system of healthcare on which our collective human dignity depends.

Several concepts were abandoned and replaced with more contemporary ones. For example, 'mastery' was felt to carry connotations of control and authority that were incompatible with contemporary notions of partnership. 'Autonomy' and 'self-regulation' were rejected on the grounds that they implied the right and authority to act independently of the wishes of the patient and the weight of available evidence, and also ran counter to the concept of team-based care. 'Privilege' was thought to be outmoded in this more egalitarian era. 'Excellence' replaced 'competence' as a higher standard to aim for. 'Judgement' was felt to better capture the processes of critical thinking that doctors apply in helping to solve patients' problems than the concept of 'the art of medicine.' The use of the term 'moral contract' added an ethical and moral dimension to the somewhat neutral concept of the 'social contract.' The concept of 'vocation' or 'calling' was felt to be worth preserving, and the Working Party was keen to stress the need for *'appropriate* accountability' to avoid creating and perpetuating a culture of blame and suspicion (*en passant,* they were refreshingly explicit about the damage to professionalism posed by the 'unrelenting focus' on targets in an environment in which, the report suggested, the 'regulatory pendulum' had swung too far and in which there was an undue focus on weakness rather than virtue). 'Altruism' was also retained as an underlying core principle, the Working Party declaring itself impressed by the trainee who said that medical practice 'requires neither humility nor altruism . . . good medical practice . . . requires both.' The report raised particular concerns about what it saw as a failure of medical leadership, alongside an increasingly neglected clinical input to management. Several other interlinked themes emerged, such as team working, appraisal, and careers, with implications for education and research. Overall the report was a commendable attempt 'to usher in a major philosophical shift in attitudes to medical practice'[24] and to put medical professionalism back on the political map.

PATIENT-CENTRED PROFESSIONALISM

The fact that the patient's interests should lie fairly and squarely at the heart of professional practice was central to the continuing debate about the meaning of 'professionalism' in the twenty-first century, and saw the emergence of a new(ish) term – 'patient-centred.' However, in the words of one author, 'Patient-centredness is becoming a widely used but poorly understood concept in medical practice. It may be most commonly understood for what it is not – technology-centred, doctor-centred, hospital-centred, disease-centred.'[25] In a thought-provoking discussion paper, Janet Askham and Alison Chisholm of the Picker Institute discussed some of the issues. 'Patient-centredness' could be one of four things:

➤ when doctors work in patients' best interests (but who defines those interests, and what happens when there is a conflict?)
➤ when doctors work in accordance with patients' *preferences* (this may be what a lot of patients want, but do people always know what is best for them?)
➤ when doctors work in partnership with patients and/or involve them closely in decisions (but how far should this go? what about power imbalances? do patients have to become 'quasi-doctors'?)
➤ when doctors take a 'patient-centred approach'[25] – that is, try to understand patients in a wider context, including their ideas, concerns, expectations and values.

However, the authors acknowledged that this may involve an altogether more complex kind of relationship which may not always either be desired by the patient, or be necessary for effective care. These four approaches, Askham and Chisholm argued, highlight some of the tensions underpinning much of the debate about the changing role of doctors, represented as a series of dichotomies. These were activity *versus* passivity, power *versus* autonomy, conflict *versus* collaboration, and emotion *versus* objectivity. Whatever the case, patient-centredness was clearly a complex and dynamic concept. After discussing contemporary roles of both 'patient' and 'doctor', and in particular areas of potential conflict, the authors concluded that patient-centredness can best be understood as doctors fulfilling their changing roles in ways that align with changing patient roles, but also working with patients and others to see whether areas of conflict can be resolved.[25]

A new version of *Good Medical Practice* was published by the GMC in 2006.[26] It included significant amendments to the original, and changes of emphasis, and was felt to offer a 'radical reinterpretation' of the underlying tenets of professionalism.[27] Two significant changes were that the document was targeted explicitly at patients as well as at doctors, and the principles themselves were no longer to be thought of as aspirational – rather, they were to be achieved and upheld by *all* doctors as a minimum standard. Although many of the changes may seem semantic (e.g. doctors and patients are now 'in partnership' and not simply in a relationship, doctors must *respond* to patient preferences and not merely recognise them, and so on), they reflected the need for the profession to embrace a new kind of professionalism. The GMC in partnership with the Medical Schools Council (MSC) has also developed a similar document for medical students and medical educators, entitled *Medical Students: Professional Behaviour and Fitness to Practise.*[28] This publication is advisory, rather than mandatory, as at the time of writing UK medical students are not registered with the GMC and therefore their conduct and any remediation is the concern of individual medical schools. (However, medical student registration is a requirement of some states in Australia.)

To end this introductory chapter we offer a final, challenging perspective on professionalism 'from outside the stockade.' Harry Cayton, the NHS's National Director for Patients and the Public (also known as 'the Patient's Tsar'), offers a different slant.[29] First, he contends, the term 'professional' now often means little other than well paid and exclusive (what's in a word?!). Furthermore, he finds a 'disturbing smugness and self-satisfaction' about contemporary definitions of professionalism. In particular, he singles out commonly stated attributes of a professional – altruism, mastery and autonomy – for criticism. Altruism is outmoded, since it allowed doctors to claim a moral superiority: 'I intend good so I do good. I do good so I am good. I am a doctor therefore I am good.'[29] Complacency may follow this certainty of goodness. Mastery implies possession of secret and exclusive knowledge that is withheld from others. Finally, autonomy, in Cayton's view the 'shibboleth' of professionalism, goes against the grain of multi-disciplinary working, teamwork and ultimately partnership. In their place he offers 'empathy', 'expertise' and 'mutuality', and suggests that the new professionalism should be redefined in terms of *relationships* – relationships with knowledge, with colleagues, with patients, with society, and with self, rather than based on individuality (i.e. focused on how a doctor behaves in relation to others, rather than what a doctor *is*).

OUTLINE OF THIS BOOK

Given the subject matter, there are invariable overlaps in material between the chapters, although each concentrates on a particular aspect of professionalism and/or professional behaviour. Chapter 2 considers in more detail the elements of a profession and the evolution of professionalism from an historical and sociological viewpoint. Chapter 3 concentrates on the code of conduct, including legal and ethical aspects of professional behaviour. Chapter 4 explores the nature of the patient–professional relationship, including boundaries and the nature of empathy. Chapter 5 focuses on professional communication in all its forms, with a discussion of confidentiality and consent. Chapter 6 explores cultural diversity and racism. Chapter 7 focuses on the professional responsibility to keep up to date (professional development), while Chapter 8 concentrates on personal development and looking after oneself. Chapter 9 explores the meaning of professional autonomy and the threat to self-regulation, and Chapters 10 and 11 focus on learning and teaching professionalism, and the necessity for assessing such learning. Chapter 12 rounds up the discussion with thoughts on social justice and professional responsibility.

REFERENCES

1 Knowles E, editor. *The Concise Oxford Dictionary of Quotations.* 4th ed. Oxford: Oxford University Press; 2001. p. 3.
2 www.gutenberg.org/etext/5070 (accessed May 2008).
3 Illich I. *Limits to Medicine: medical nemesis – the expropriation of health.* New ed. London: Boyars; 1976.
4 Hilton SR, Slotnick HB. Proto-professionalism: how professionalisation occurs across the continuum of medical education. *Med Educ.* 2005; **39**: 58–65.
5 http://en.wikipedia.org/wiki/Professional_foul (accessed May 2008).
6 General Medical Council. *Tomorrow's Doctors. Recommendations on undergraduate medical education.* London: General Medical Council; 1993.
7 Calman K. The profession of medicine. *BMJ.* 1994; **309**: 1140–44.
8 Smith R. Medicine's core values. *BMJ.* 1994; **309**: 1247–8.
9 British Medical Association. *Core Values for the Medical Profession in the 21st Century: report of conference.* London: British Medical Association; 1995.
10 General Medical Council. *Duties of a Doctor.* London: General Medical Council; 1995.
11 General Medical Council. *Good Medical Practice.* London: General Medical Council; 1995.
12 www.bristol-inquiry.org.uk/final_report/index.htm (accessed May 2008).
13 Irvine D. *The Doctor's Tale.* Oxford: Radcliffe Medical Press; 2003.
14 Smith R. All changed, changed utterly. *BMJ.* 1998; **316**: 1917–18.
15 www.abim.org/pdf/publications/professionalism.pdf (accessed May 2008).

16 Swick HM. Toward a normative definition of medical professionalism. *Acad Med.* 2000; **75**: 612–16.

17 Project of the ABIM Foundation, ACP-ASIM Foundation, and European Federation of Internal Medicine. Medical professionalism in the new millennium: a physician charter. *Ann Intern Med.* 2002; **136**: 243–6.

18 http://meds.queensu.ca/medicine/obgyn/pdf/CanMEDS.overview.pdf (accessed May 2008).

19 Cruess SR, Cruess RL. Professionalism must be taught. *BMJ.* 1997; **315**: 1674–7.

20 Novack DH, Suchman AL, Clark W *et al.* for the Working Group on Promoting Physician Personal Awareness, American Academy on Physician and Patient. Calibrating the physician. Personal awareness and effective patient care. *JAMA.* 1997; **278**: 502–9.

21 Faulkner LR, McCurdy RL. Teaching medical students social responsibility. The right thing to do. *Acad Med.* 2000; **75**: 346–50.

22 O'Neill O. *A Question of Trust. The BBC Reith Lectures 2002.* Cambridge: Cambridge University Press; 2002.

23 Rosen R, Dewar S. *On Being a Doctor. Redefining medical professionalism for better patient care.* London: King's Fund; 2004.

24 Royal College of Physicians. *Doctors in Society. Medical professionalism in a changing world. Report of a Working Party of the RCP.* London: Royal College of Physicians; 2005.

25 Askham J, Chisholm A. *Patient-Centred Medical Professionalism: towards an agenda for research and action;* www.pickereurope.org/Filestore/RapidResponse/pcpconcepts-report-PDF.pdf (accessed May 2008).

26 General Medical Council. *Good Medical Practice.* London: General Medical Council; 2006.

27 Horton R, Gilmore I. The evolving doctor. *Lancet.* 2006; **368**: 1750–51.

28 Medical Schools' Council and General Medical Council. *Medical Students: professional behaviour and fitness to practise.* London: Medical Schools' Council and General Medical Council; 2007.

29 www.asme.org.uk/conf_courses/2005/docs_pix/04_28_cayton.pdf (accessed May 2008).

CHAPTER 2

Learning from history

This chapter explores:
- the elements of a profession and their evolution
- the professionalisation of medicine
- the Hippocratic Oath
- the history of certification and licensing
- the birth of the General Medical Council
- the National Health Service
- the Conservative government and the internal market
- the Labour government and commissioning
- the sociologists' viewpoint
- the healer versus the professional.

> Roughly it may be said professions in England are valued according to their stability, their remunerativeness, their influence and their recognition by the State.
>
> *Escott, 1885*[1]

> Professionalism is most in need of defence in the case of medicine, for the latter's crisis continues and is intensifying.
>
> *Freidson, 1994*[2]

A discussion of the history of professionalism hinges on the many definitions of the word as detailed in Chapter 1. The word 'profession' itself comes from the Latin *profiteri* (to avow or confess). By the mid-seventeenth century it was being applied to three main occupations of university graduates – divinity, law and physic[3] – although all of the elements later considered to be necessary for a profession did not exist at that time. Thus, for example, a monk 'professed' when he took his final vows and entered a monastery for life. 'Professor' as an English word was first used in Henry VIII's reign to mean a public teacher.[4] Doctor, from the Latin *docere* (to teach), meant a university teacher and dates from about 500 years earlier than this. It was first applied to a doctor of medicine in Salerno around 1221.[5]

THE EVOLUTION OF THE PROFESSIONS

The American scholar Eliot Freidson, the doyen of sociologist writers on the professions, believes that we should not attempt to treat 'profession' as a generic concept, but rather as a changing historical concept, and furthermore as a concept whose roots lie in Anglo-American industrial nations.[2] Therefore the nature of professionalism is also open to interpretation depending on the era under consideration. It is difficult to do justice to the many and varied arguments about this topic in one chapter; only a flavour of the debate is possible with the highlighting of important dates and commentaries. However, at this point we may list the six elements of a profession that appear most commonly in the literature:

➤ the presence of skill based on specialist knowledge
➤ provision of training and education
➤ the means of testing for competence
➤ organisation of members
➤ adherence to a code of conduct
➤ the provision of an altruistic service not just for financial reward.[6]

(Compare these elements defined in 1972 to those of the GMC from 1994 in Chapter 1.) The development of professions with all of these elements occurred in the Victorian era in the UK. When considering the history of professionalism, while professions other than medicine should not be neglected, according to one commentator the medical profession holds one of the most privileged, autonomous positions in the marketplace, with perhaps only law occupying a similar niche.[7]

Underpinning these six requirements is the fundamental characteristic of professional autonomy, equated to self-governance and self-regulation: 'the professional organisation rather than the society or the client defines the nature of the expected service . . . because the profession claims to be the only legitimate arbiter of improper performance of service. Every profession has a professional ideology which explains why professional autonomy is not desired out of self-interest, but is a requirement for offering the best possible service in the public interest.'[8] This autonomy extends to defining the educational needs of members, the licensing structure, the setting and enforcing of technical expertise and the ethical code, and the granting and revoking of licenses to practise. Professional autonomy is covered in greater detail in Chapter 9.

Much has been written about the nature of the professions, and professionalism and its development, particularly from a sociological perspective. Historians and sociologists have various and differing viewpoints about the impact of professionalism on individuals and populations; interested readers will be able to make use of the references to study the issues in more detail. The history of the medical profession may be simply stated as a series of landmark events, but the history of the analysis of the nature of professionalism itself is also interesting and worthy of consideration. Medical writers and educators tend to view professionalism as a 'good thing.' A recent Dutch study sought to clarify the elements of medical professionalism. The long list generated included only positive aspects, such as altruism, accountability, respect, integrity, lifelong learning, and so on.[9] Yet the social scientists are far more critical of the subject, and write at length about the negative aspects of monopoly, elitism and self-regulation. For example, Freidson believes that professions, including medicine, often use their monopoly to improve their economic interests more than is necessary, and are reluctant to judge the performance of their members sufficiently critically.[2] However, he also warns against weakening the desirable elements of professionalism.

The sociologists Gerstl and Jacobs believe that the processes of professionalisation, de-professionalisation and re-professionalisation are cyclical. In 1976 they wrote that society was in a stage of advanced elitist professionalisation but, should history repeat itself, it was also on the verge of de-professionalisation.[10] In the opinion of some commentators their prediction has come true, as during the last quarter of the twentieth century the medical profession underwent a period of intense scrutiny and doctors' autonomy was challenged due to several forces that will be discussed later in this chapter. However, the extent of this de-professionalisation, if it happened at all, is debatable, as we shall see. In particular, defining cycles of 'professional dominance', 'proletarianisation', 'de-professionalisation' and 'corporatisation', as political commentators are liable to do, has been criticised as ignoring the dynamic relationship between the professions and society.[11] It is obvious that a study of professionalism involves a whole new jargon. The challenge is to present and discuss what is relevant to medical practice now. Some understanding of history is always important for contemporary life.

This chapter concentrates mainly on the change in the status of medical practice in the UK, although there are some references to the USA. There are obvious differences between the two countries, but also a greater similarity than between, for example, the UK and parts of Europe that retain a centralist state control of the professions.

HIPPOCRATES AND THE GREEK TRADITION

As mentioned above, members of a profession differ from those outside it by virtue of their knowledge and skills acquired through specialist training. Hippocrates, who lived and practised around 420 BCE, is generally credited with being the 'father of medicine.' Although details of his life are patchy, we do know that his birthplace, the island of Cos, was home to a society of physicians. Several such closed societies or guilds existed in Greece at that time, named after the demigod, and son of Apollo, Aesculapius (or Asclepius). The Coan society set up a school complete with library to train medical apprentices in observation, note keeping and the art of diagnosis.[12] It is of course from Cos that the Hippocratic Oath derives. This is an oath containing an ethical code that doctors professed in some form for the following two millennia. One version is given in Box 2.1. Modern versions also exist which take into account changes in medical and ethical practice over the centuries. But how many doctors do 'profess' such an oath these days?

BOX 2.1 THE HIPPOCRATIC OATH, TRANSLATED FROM THE GREEK BY LUDWIG EDELSTEIN[13]

I swear by Apollo Physician and Asclepius and Hygieia and Panaceia and all the gods and goddesses, making them my witnesses, that I will fulfil according to my ability and judgment this oath and this covenant: To hold him who has taught me this art as equal to my parents and to live my life in partnership with him, and if he is in need of money to give him a share of mine, and to regard his offspring as equal to my brothers in male lineage and to teach them this art – if they desire to learn it – without fee and covenant; to give a share of precepts and oral instruction and all the other learning to my sons and to the sons of him who has instructed me and to pupils who have signed the covenant and have taken an oath according to the medical law, but no one else. I will apply dietetic measures for the benefit of the sick according to my ability and judgment; I will keep them from harm and injustice. I will neither give a deadly drug to anybody who asked for it, nor will I make a suggestion to this effect. Similarly I will not give to a woman an abortive remedy. In purity and holiness I will guard my life and my art. I will not use the knife, not even on sufferers from stone, but will withdraw in favour of such men as are engaged in this work. Whatever houses I may visit, I will come for the benefit of the sick, remaining free of all intentional injustice, of all mischief and in particular of sexual relations with both female and male persons, be they free or slaves. What I may see or hear in the course of the treatment or even outside of the treatment in regard to the life of men, which on no account one must spread abroad, I will keep to myself, holding such things shameful to be spoken about. If I fulfil this oath and do not violate it, may it be granted to me to enjoy life and art, being honoured with fame among all men for all time to come; if I transgress it and swear falsely, may the opposite of all this be my lot.

Although the Hippocratic Oath contains elements of the doctor as an altruistic ethical healer, it also reinforces the idea of medicine as a 'closed shop' and encourages patronage. Education and support are available to members of the profession, those linked by their taking of the oath, and to no one else. The mysteries of health and healing are only to be known by the privileged few. Penalties for transgression are hinted at – the gods are asked not to look favourably on someone who does not uphold the high standards of the group. A possible legacy of the oath is the division of practitioners into physicians and surgeons within the Western medical tradition. Although doctors qualify these days with joint certification in both medicine and surgery, this division does perhaps partly account for the lack of an holistic approach to patient care. Modern undergraduate medical curricula usually attempt to integrate the teaching of internal medicine and surgery, but hospital posts do not always reflect such education. Increasing specialisation in a doctor's later career also tends to lead to a lack of continuity in a patient's care – he sees one doctor for his heart problems, one for his asthma, one for his hernia, and so on. Threats to the existence of the generalist in medicine may exacerbate this problem.

CONTROL AND CERTIFICATION

With the rise of the university system in Europe occurring in parallel with the learning of the art of medicine via apprenticeship, the states began to intervene in the licensing of doctors. In England, the first medical act was passed by Henry VIII in 1511–1512, making it unlawful to practise either as a physician or as a surgeon unless one possessed a university degree or a license issued by a bishop, the latter being conferred after examination by a panel of experts. The aim of the act was to reduce the numbers of 'quacks' and untrained practitioners who advised and/or dispensed treatments without acceptable training. However, the act met its aim too successfully, and within 25 years there were not enough licensed people to meet the public's demand. The 1542 Act therefore recognised the expertise of lay persons who had such knowledge of herbs and roots that they could treat illness without formal training. However, only the licensed doctors could charge a fee for advice – an incentive for those who could afford it to become part of the recognised professional body.

In the sixteenth and seventeenth centuries physicians had university degrees, obtained through study of the classics but often with no practical experience, while surgeons trained via apprenticeship. The third group of aspiring medical practitioners were the apothecaries. Apothecaries were tradesmen like the surgeons, allied as they were to grocers and spicers, selling foodstuffs as well as drugs. To comply with the 1542 Act they only charged for the cost of the medicine dispensed, and were therefore an affordable option for the poorer classes of society.

The notion of a strictly tripartite hierarchy of medical practice, with the gentlemen physicians at the top, the manual surgeons in the middle and the tradesmen apothecaries at the bottom, has been challenged by the late medical historian and prolific writer Roy Porter.[14] Although this traditional picture reflected reality to some extent in London, where the three groups were licensed and regulated by the College of Physicians, the Corporation of Surgeons and the Society of Apothecaries, respectively, the situation in the rest of the country was very different. Here all manner of medical practitioners pursued the public to make a living – their success depended on satisfaction of their patients rather then their peers.[14] These practitioners included some physicians (although few were university educated), many surgeons, apothecaries and apothecary-surgeons, as well as large numbers of 'Mountebanks, Quacksalvers, Empiricks',[15] all competing in the same market. (There are some parallels with the current situation with regard to practitioners of complementary medicine, who hold a bewildering variety of qualifications to confuse the patient.)

The eighteenth century was a time of great change. The Enlightenment and scientific discoveries allied to the foundation of hospitals in the large centres of population in Great Britain led to a change in medical education and a call for a new system of licensing for medical practitioners. There was a growing theoretical knowledge base and a greater understanding of anatomy that could be taught, although this knowledge did not translate into better healthcare and prognoses. Due to the growing population, once again there was a shortage of trained doctors. Social class and wealth now became an important determinant of healthcare. The rich (the aristocracy and the new industrialists) were treated by university-trained physicians, and demand for such gentleman professionals could not be met, while the less wealthy looked to the tradesmen surgeons and apothecaries for healthcare. Physicians wrote prescriptions in Latin, which were dispensed by apothecaries (forerunners of the modern pharmacist), and they charged large fees. Surgeons spoke in the vernacular and were more affordable. However, there was a market for regular medical care across the whole range of social classes, with patients consulting medical practitioners for both serious illnesses and more minor self-limiting conditions.[16]

The three branches of health practitioners could not agree on the limits of their own expertise, but all wanted recognition of their right to practise medicine. In 1815, Parliament passed the Apothecaries Act, which forced a major change in licensing. Under this act, all new apothecaries in England and Wales had to serve a 5-year apprenticeship and be examined and then licensed by the Society of Apothecaries. In theory the latter had the power to prosecute anyone who practised without their licence, but in practice they did not do so if men possessed qualifications from either the universities or the Royal College of Physicians (founded in 1518 as the London College of Physicians). The Royal College of Surgeons (founded in 1800) allied itself with the apothecaries, and thus the majority of licences issued in the mid-nineteenth century were joint MRCS (Membership of the Royal College of Surgeons) and LSA (Licentiate of the Society of Apothecaries).

Along with this reform of certification, medical education was being scrutinised and improved. Eventually, in 1854, a university medical degree became formally acceptable as a license to practise medicine. The Medical Act of 1858 simplified matters by placing all of the different licensing bodies under the control of the General Council of Medical Education and Registration, the agency that later became the General Medical Council (GMC). The GMC compiled and kept a register of qualified doctors as well as defining what constituted appropriate courses for medical training. However, it did not abolish the different ways of achieving a licence (unlike the USA, which developed a single qualification – the MD). The main remit of the GMC was to protect patients from unlicensed practitioners, although it could only prosecute those practitioners who posed as medically qualified. However, the GMC also had a remit to protect the qualified medical practitioner. The tension between these two functions of protecting doctors and protecting patients fuels much of the current debate about professionalism and the future role of the GMC. Through the development of its ethical code, the GMC also raised the status of doctors, and indeed it is from the time of founding of the GMC that we may say that medicine became a true profession, as opposed to a trade.

THE PROFESSIONALISATION OF MEDICINE

The 1858 Medical Act allowed for the self-regulation of the profession, relatively free from lay and government control. The GMC was given a virtual monopoly to provide medical services, control medical training, restrict recruitment by means of the medical register, and discipline doctors whose behaviour was considered inappropriate.[17] By virtue of registration with the GMC a person could demonstrate their qualification to practise medicine. 'Unqualified' practitioners such as herbalists and homeopaths could ply their trade, but they were unable to provide state certification, and were further disadvantaged by their lack of state legitimacy and thus status.

One intriguing aspect of the Act is the institutionalisation, and subsequent professionalisation, of the orthodox biomedical perspective of the Western medical tradition, and the marginalisation of what is now called alternative or complementary medicine. After the Act there was only one approved supply of medical services, whereas previously there had been competition feeding this universal need for healing. There are a number of sociological theories to account for this development. The functionalist argument that only the emerging scientific medicine was effective in treating disease has been criticised because the main advances in diagnosis and pharmacology did not take place until much later than the mid-nineteenth century.[18] Indeed bloodletting was still a widespread practice in 1858.

Another effect of the 1858 Act, and the subsequent Medical Act of 1886 that required doctors to be examined in midwifery as well as in medicine and surgery, was to reduce the number of doctors practising in the UK. This consequence, coupled with the increasing demand for medical services from a growing urban population, led to the enhanced prosperity of doctors around the turn of the century. The Acts also led to the abolishment of the apprenticeship method of medical education and the establishment of the university- and hospital-based courses that are the norm to the present day. This concentration of a cohort of medical students in one place to study assisted the further development of a common professional identity. Such professional socialisation has been blamed for the distancing of students from the influence of the public, and thus 'enhancing the power of the profession against outsiders.'[18]

Of course people did not immediately entrust themselves to only one brand of medical management. Custom and income were important factors in deciding where one went for medical advice. For example, patent medicines that were sold by advertising in papers and on the streets were very much in demand until the early twentieth century. Larson suggests that two factors in the public's increasing patronage of licensed practitioners were the ability to consult a doctor in private about personal problems, and the increasing number of public hospitals, provided by the state, which were staffed by state-approved practitioners.[19]

BOX 2.2 DATES IN THE PROFESSIONALISATION OF MEDICINE

1511–12	First Medical Act	License needed to practise physic or surgery
1518	College of Physicians founded	(Became Royal in 1551)
1542	Medical Act	Recognition of lay expertise 'Quacks' Charter'
1617	Society of Apothecaries becomes free from grocers' guild	
1703	Rose decision	Right of apothecaries to act as doctors
1800	Company of Surgeons becomes Royal College of Surgeons	
1815	Apothecaries' Act	Licensing and apprenticeship mandatory
1816	Foundation of Worcester Medical and Surgical Society (becomes British Medical Association in 1855)	
1854	Medical degree acceptable as license to practise medicine	
1858	General Council of Medical Education and Registration (establishes right to self-regulation, professionalisation of medicine)	

These hospitals also required staffing by personnel other than doctors. At this point in history neither the state nor the medical profession had an official method of managing this growing allied workforce. However, they had a joint interest in controlling these newly emerging occupations and continuing to exclude certain practitioners.[20] While midwives, nurses and dentists became state regulated in the early decades of the twentieth century, alternative practitioners remained outside the medical mainstream. However, the latter were still able to practise, although they were not registered. The GMC had the power to remove from its register any doctor who worked with an unrecognised practitioner of any kind. Although Larkin (of Sheffield Hallam University) feels that this exclusion was the result of the opposition of doctors to any form of dilution of their privileges, the GMC presented things in a different light. Rather than being self-interested behaviour, the blocking of official recognition of herbalists and osteopaths was said to be a way of keeping the public out of the harmful range of unauthorised practitioners. Although some doctors were prepared to agree that osteopathy had considerable though limited usefulness, they thought that it should only be allowed when subordinated to medical control.[20] Similar limitations were imposed in the USA.

Important dates and events in the professionalisation of medical practice are listed in Box 2.2.

THE NATIONAL HEALTH SERVICE

The Beveridge Report of 1942 proposed a comprehensive National Health Service (NHS), including general practice and hospital treatment, free at the point of delivery, for the whole of Great Britain. The service would be funded by social insurance contributions covering all income groups. The report did not rule out private medical practice coexisting with the state-financed system. The British Medical Association agreed with the proposal on the condition that doctors would be involved in negotiating the character, terms and conditions of service within the new service.[12] Doctors who were registered with the GMC would charge no fees within this health service, but unorthodox practitioners would not be available to patients under the state insurance scheme and thus would become exclusively private practitioners.

As noted above, professionals are expected to demonstrate a certain degree of altruism and not to work solely for financial gain. Yet at the time of the creation of the NHS in 1948, many doctors opposed the move towards a state-sponsored service, not only because they were afraid of losing their autonomy, but also because they would lose the right to set their own fees. Aneurin Bevan, the Labour MP responsible for the initial development of the NHS, famously said that he enticed doctors to work within the new service because 'I stuffed their mouths with gold.'[21] Hospital doctors received salaries based on their seniority, while general practitioners were paid mainly through capitation fees – that is, on the basis of the number of patients registered with them as providers of medical services. Doctors in the USA saw such state control and bureaucracy as de-professionalisation. However, in fact the state financing of British healthcare led to an increased income for doctors as well as improvements in status and power because of the monopoly that they enjoyed.[22]

The British welfare state, of which the NHS is a major component, was developed on the principles that certain sections of the population (the elderly, unemployed and chronically ill) would not be able to pay for appropriate health and social care, and that such care was not a market commodity. Both the Labour and Conservative parties agreed on this, and also that healthcare should be provided by the state, for over 20 years following the birth of the NHS. Central to these principles was that the allocation of resources would be delegated by the state to the medical profession. Doctors were given a key role in identifying people who required services, thus ensuring that the welfare state was a 'professional state.'[23] This was acceptable to the populace, who viewed doctors as neutral agents, acting in the best interests of patients, who would ensure equitable and efficient use of public funds.[23] In 1951 the sociologist Talcot Parsons stressed the suitability of the medical profession for this role, given their lack of self-interest compared with profit-making organisations and 'big business.' For this reason he also believed that healthcare could not be delivered within a market framework, with doctors competing against each other.[24] However, Margaret Thatcher (UK Prime Minister from 1979 to 1990) was to have other ideas.

Other countries have dealt with the provision of medical services for their citizens in a variety of ways, ranging from the services being free at the point of delivery (such as the NHS) to a completely private system where patients pay for their healthcare when necessary. Most countries fall somewhere between these two systems, and have a public health service funded by taxation running alongside a private service funded by medical insurance or fees paid directly by the patient. In the UK, doctors working for the NHS are, on the whole, not allowed to charge patients. However, British doctors may work within both the public and private sectors, and in the latter charge fees.

THE INTERNAL MARKET: THE NATIONAL HEALTH SERVICE IN THE 1990s

Two Austrian analysts had doubts about the benefits of living within a welfare state. The right-wing economist Friedrich Hayek (1899–1992) wrote as early as 1944 that such a state created a dependency in its subjects that could be likened to slavery. The state provision of healthcare destroyed a population's ability to look after itself.[25] Thirty years later, Ivan Illich (1926–2002), whose life's work concentrated on dissecting the institutional structures of industrialised societies, such as schooling, transport and – perhaps most notoriously – health, criticised the monopoly enjoyed by the medical profession. According to Illich this monopoly controlled both the demand for and the supply of health services, leading to the medicalisation of people's social and personal problems.[26] Illich is of course noted for his analysis of the lack of impact of medical advances on the health of nations, major improvements in health being the result of improved living conditions and sanitation.

When Margaret Thatcher's Conservative Party came to power in 1979, expenditure on the health service was placing a strain on the economy. Doctors appeared to have sole control of health spending, with minimal accountability. High-technology medicine was consuming costs at the expense of more effective services such as preventive medicine and general practice. Moreover, care of the more vulnerable sections of society, such as the elderly and disabled, was seen as a less glamorous alternative on which to base one's medical career, leading to neglect in these areas. Something had to be done. The welfare state could not be dismantled, as this would be too unpopular a solution. However, some kind of hybrid between the NHS and the free market was seen as a possible compromise.

The 1989 White Paper *Working for Patients*[27] and the resulting 1990 National Health Service and Community Care Act created an internal market in healthcare. The aim was to give patients, now seen as 'consumers', increased information about and choice of health provision. The terminology of this change is interesting. Unlike other market situations, the patient-consumer was not called a purchaser. Purchasers (GPs) were still within the profession, buying services with 'funds' on behalf of their registered patients from the providers, such as hospitals and allied health professionals. This gave power – albeit limited – to those general practitioners who became 'fundholders', but at the same time they were to be held accountable for how they spent their resources.

Fundholding led to disagreements within the profession. Not all general practices were eligible to become fundholders. Moreover, not all GPs agreed with the principle of the internal market thus created. Patients of those GPs who did receive a budget theoretically had more choice with regard to where they were referred for hospital and other services. However, in practice it was the GPs who decided where to place their contracts and purchase such services. Many doctors felt that this process created a two-tier service; fundholding practices had greater flexibility in what they were able to offer their patients.[28] For example, some GPs used their budget to employ physiotherapists and counselling services directly. However, any money in the fund that was not spent within a financial year could be used by the doctors to improve their premises – premises that were often owned by the doctors themselves in the first place. This money could therefore be used to enhance the individual wealth of the GPs. Patients from fundholding practices were able to jump the queue on waiting lists.

THE NATIONAL HEALTH SERVICE UNDER NEW LABOUR

The Labour party came to power in 1997 under the leadership of Tony Blair, whose electoral success was based on a revamping of the historical socialist principles of the party now branded as 'New Labour.' Within two years the Labour Government had abolished fundholding and the internal market because they disapproved of competition within the NHS. The 1999 Health Act created a primary care-led health service with the establishment of primary care trusts (PCTs). More than 300 of these district-based bodies commission services from hospitals. However, recent developments mean that, for example, refurbishment of premises may now be carried out in (potentially) lucrative partnership with the private sector through the Private Finance Initiative (PFI). GPs once again are being invited to become practice-based commissioners, with the promise that they will be able to keep 50% of any savings that they make from their new-look 'funds.' Practices will thus benefit financially if they send fewer patients for investigations or make fewer referrals to specialists. Plans are also being drawn up at Government level for commercial providers to take over primary and community care.

Since its inception the NHS has undergone many reorganisations, and it appears to lurch from one crisis to another. Clinicians often disagree with politicians and managers on the best ways to deliver quality and safe patient care. In 2008 it is being questioned whether the health service is truly national as the governments of the four home nations (England, Wales, Scotland and Northern Island) choose different priorities for funding, and embrace or shun the market-based reforms. In Scotland, ministers are putting their faith in 'professionals' and clinical networks of specialist doctors to allocate resources and deliver services.[29]

WRITING ABOUT THE PROFESSIONS

Interest in the history of the professions began to develop about a century ago. Notable works were written by the socialists Sidney and Beatrice Webb[30] (who were also the founders of the *New Statesman*), and by the radical RH Tawney.[31] In his book published in 1928, Carr-Saunders wrote that one of the common features of all professions is a universal rule against advertising.[32] (This rule is not so universal now, with doctors certainly advertising their *private* services on the Internet and in glossy brochures.) At this time the concept of 'profession' was largely taken for granted, and it was not until the expansion of academic sociology in the USA after the Second World War that the theory of professionalism began to be considered.[2]

Freidson notes that, although writers in the 1940s and 1950s recognised and criticised the deficiencies of the professions, particularly with regard to their self-interest, on the whole their views were positive. The knowledge and skills of professional people and the mainly altruistic way in which they worked were highlighted at this time. Parsons indeed wrote that the professions were creating a new form of social structure that was reducing the political authoritarianism of the capitalist state, with its focus on profit and exploitation.[24] However, from the 1960s, in both the USA and the UK, the professions began to be attacked. Their cultural and political influence was cited and their roots in the class system were identified.[33] Attention was drawn to the financial rewards of a professional career. Professionalisation was defined as 'an attempt to translate one order of scarce resources – knowledge and skills – into another – social and economic rewards.'[19] This process created a monopoly in the medical profession by the control of licensing, and accentuated the role of education in subsequent social inequality.[19]

An example of the extent of negative feeling 'against the professions' can be found in a publication by a member of the Libertarian Alliance based in London. In 1983 he cited lack of competition between members of the profession, self-regulation and state sponsorship as reasons why, rather than the public being protected, the profession is itself protected against public complaints. Although the effectiveness of the argument is reduced somewhat by the false statement that all doctors must be members of the British Medical Association (rather than, as is the case, registered with the General Medical Council), the publication does raise questions about the way in which doctors practise. In particular, one criticism was the lack of feedback between the public and the profession.[34]

THE HEALER VERSUS THE PROFESSIONAL

In an article published in the *British Medical Journal* in 1997, two Canadian professors, Sylvia and Richard Cruess, wrote that doctors are simultaneously both healers and professionals.[35] This is a thought-provoking distinction that may be related to the doctor–patient relationship in which the professional role leads to an institutional bond between doctor and patient, while the healer role involves a more humane dimension.[36] The institutional bond arises because the role of the state is symbiotic with the role of the professional – what Klein calls the 'politics of the double bed.'[37] This tension is apparent throughout the history of the professionalisation of medicine, with altruism, resource allocation, rationing and individual versus public health priorities competing for the doctor's attention. We may also consider the important concepts of doctor-centredness (and paternalism) and patient-centredness.

While Sylvia and Richard Cruess listed the attributes of the healer and the professional in a workshop presented at the Tenth Ottawa Conference on Medical Education in 2002[38] (*see* Box 2.3), they did not themselves dissect the nature of these attributes with regard to the change in focus of medical practice since the eighteenth century. Indeed most medical commentators on professionalism write from the perspective that it is a principle that should be pursued, and that it is desirable from the point of view of both the doctor and the patient.[39] However, it is possible that this is not the case.

BOX 2.3 ATTRIBUTES OF THE HEALER AND THE PROFESSIONAL[38]

Healer	*Healer and professional*	*Professional*
Caring and compassionate	Competent	Self-regulated
Insightful	Committed	Responsible:
Open	Autonomous	to society
Respectful of healing	Altruistic	to profession
Respectful of patient	Honest	Team worker
Not distracted	Moral and ethical	

The medical profession adopted the biomedical tradition, and this circumstance has been blamed for the rise of medical paternalism and the disempowerment of patients.[40] With scientific progress in medicine and the change from consultations at the bedside (i.e. at home) to consultations in hospital, the 'sick man' and his illness story disappeared and the 'patient' – a pathological body studded with lesions – appeared.[41] The biomedical model has been held responsible for divorcing medicine from the social fabric of patients' lives.[42]

As early as the eighteenth century, Thomas Percival (1740–1804) advocated reinforcing paternalism, especially with regard to poorer and charity patients, although he admitted that adopting an authoritarian stance towards paying patients might be more difficult.[43] Percival's *Handbook of Medical Ethics* gave guidance as to how doctors should behave towards patients, and is really more concerned with professional etiquette than with what we would today term 'medical ethics.' Parsons viewed the doctor as an agent of social control, allowing (or not) the patient's continuation of the sick role by the doctor's power of sick certification and social sanctioning. In Parson's analysis, the doctor–patient relationship is a formal and distant one. The doctor expects the patient 'to obey' the doctor without question.[24]

We could think of the 'healer' as person-centred and the 'professional' as doctor-centred. The movement in the latter half of the twentieth century to a person-centred approach in consultations, together with patient partnership and shared decision making, could therefore be said by advocates of medical power to be de-professionalising medicine – and similarly the increasing presence of lay people on the GMC, the involvement of the public in decisions relating to National Health Service policy, the assessment of doctors by 'real' and 'simulated' patients, and the concept of the 'expert patient.'[44,45]

	Goals	Power base	Possible adverse outcomes
Doctor as healer	To provide best possible care for sick patients To develop the evidence base of medicine	Doctors Working towards doctor–patient partnership	Rationing Imbalance of individual versus population needs Wants versus needs of patients
Doctor as professional	To preserve professional autonomy To increase wealth To increase prestige	Doctors	State interference State employment State regulation
State	To provide effective healthcare at lowest possible cost	State	Demoralisation of profession Discontent of patients Depersonalised care
Patient	To be healthy Effective, prompt and convenient healthcare when ill	Patient groups Working towards doctor–patient partnership	Medicalisation of 'normal' function Iatrogenic illness Consumerism Over-reliance on medical care Move towards complementary practitioners
Corporations (pharmaceutical, etc.)	To increase profits To advance the scientific basis of medicine Marketing of new products Cornering markets Creating new markets	Shareholders Some state control	Medicalisation of 'normal' function Iatrogenic illness Ever increasing costs of healthcare Postcode prescribing Doctors dependent on corporations' interests Influence on clinical decisions

FIGURE 2.1 Goals and challenges of different stakeholders.

The 'doctor as healer' wants the best for his or her patient, but the 'doctor as professional' has to be aware of the needs of the population, the demands on an already stretched health service, and the increasing costs to taxpayers of advances in medical science. The doctor as professional has to consider rationing and prioritisation of medical services. In the UK, demand is controlled to some extent by waiting lists. There is a danger that the self-interest of a given medical specialty, in enhancing its own reputation by introducing new, expensive and perhaps untested techniques, will lead to an imbalance in service provided in different parts of the country. 'Postcode rationing' or inequality of access to certain drugs or procedures has been a feature of the UK system that has angered patient groups, excited politicians, and offered the media much fodder, again leading to a call for greater involvement of professionals in health service planning (as appears to be happening in Scotland, as mentioned above). Figure 2.1 compares the goals and challenges of different stakeholders with regard to the practice of medicine in the UK.

THE AMERICAN EXPERIENCE

The recent history of the medical profession in the USA has parallels with the situation in the UK, although it is distinctly different. After reaching perhaps its heyday in the 1960s, many aspects of the way in which the profession organised itself, such as medical school selection, accreditation and licensure, and professional bodies, came under close scrutiny because of increasing medical fees. In the 1970s the Federal Trades Commission decided that such practices were restrictive, and described the medical profession somewhat simplistically as 'sinister actors who restrained competition unfairly in order to lock in high medical fees.'[46] The rise of managed care from the 1980s onwards following the decision by the federal government, with the support of the profession, not to introduce universal healthcare insurance, left the medical profession 'out on a limb to be picked over by creative corporations.'[46] This appears to have isolated the profession and put it in conflict with both the government and commerce (as represented by managed care), ultimately to no one's benefit, least of all that of the patients.

SUMMARY

The six elements that may be said to constitute a profession came together for medicine in the mid-nineteenth century. Although doctors themselves on the whole think that professionalism is a good thing, this is not the view of sociologists, some of whom see the medical profession as an elite, self-regulating group. The UK National Health Service is a state-sponsored institution that allows doctors a monopoly of care, even within an internal-market situation. The professional role of doctors may cause tension with their more traditional role as healers.

REFERENCES

1 Escott THS. *England: her people, polity and pursuits.* New York: Henry Holt & Co; 1885.
2 Freidson E. *Professionalism Reborn. Theory, prophecy and policy.* Cambridge: Polity Press; 1994.
3 Pest W. *The Professions in Early Modern England.* London: Croom Helm; 1987.
4 Soanes C, Stevenson A, editors. *Oxford Dictionary of English.* 2nd ed. Oxford: Oxford University Press; 2003.
5 Guthrie D. *A History of Medicine.* London: Thomas Nelson; 1945.
6 Johnson TJ. *Professions and Power.* London: Macmillan Press Limited; 1972.
7 Macdonald K. *The Sociology of the Professions.* London: Sage; 1995.
8 Daniels AK. How free should professions be? In: Freidson E, editor. *The Professions and Their Prospects.* Thousand Oaks, CA: Sage; 1971. pp. 39–57.
9 Van de Camp K, Vernooij-Dassen MJFJ, Grol RPTM *et al.* How to conceptualise professionalism: a qualitative study. *Med Teach.* 2004; **26:** 696–702.
10 Gerstl J, Jacobs G. *Professions for the People. The politics of skills.* New York: New Schenkman Publishing Company; 1976.
11 Light D. Countervailing powers. A framework for professions in transition. In: Johnson T, Larkin G, Saks M, editors. *Health Professions and the State in Europe.* London: Routledge; 1995. pp. 25–41.
12 Cartwright FF. *A Social History of Medicine.* London: Longman; 1977.
13 Edelstein L. *The Hippocratic Oath: text, translation, and interpretation.* Baltimore, MD: Johns Hopkins Press; 1943.
14 Porter R, Porter D. *Patients' Progress. Doctors and doctoring in eighteenth-century England.* Cambridge: Polity Press; 1989.
15 Burton R. *The Anatomy of Melancholy.* New York: Tudor Publishing Company; 1948 (first published in London in 1621).
16 Loudon I. *Medical Care and the General Practitioner 1750–1850.* Oxford: Clarendon Press; 1986.
17 Stacey M. *Regulating British Medicine: the General Medical Council.* Chichester: John Wiley & Sons; 1992.
18 Saks M. *Orthodox and Alternative Medicine. Politics, professionalisation and health care.* London: Continuum; 2003.
19 Larson MS. *The Rise of Professionalism: a sociological analysis.* Berkeley, CA: University of California Press; 1977.
20 Larkin G. State control and health professions. In: Johnson T, Larkin G, Saks M, editors. *Health Professions and the State in Europe.* London: Routledge; 1995. pp. 45–54.
21 Knowles E, editor. *The Concise Oxford Dictionary of Quotations.* 4th ed. Oxford: Oxford University Press; 2001.

22 Berlant JL. *Profession and Monopoly: a study of medicine in the United States and Great Britain.* Berkeley, CA: University of California Press; 1975.

23 Alaszewski A. Restructuring health and welfare professions in the United Kingdom. In: Johnson T, Larkin G, Saks M, editors. *Health Professions and the State in Europe.* London: Routledge; 1995. pp. 55–74.

24 Parsons T. *The Social System.* London: Routledge and Kegan Paul; 1951.

25 Hayek F. *The Road to Serfdom.* London: Routledge; 1944.

26 Illich I. *Limits to Medicine: medical nemesis – the expropriation of health.* Harmondsworth: Penguin; 1976.

27 Department of Health. *Working for Patients.* London: HMSO; 1989.

28 Peacock S. *Experiences with the UK National Health Service Reforms: a case of the infernal market?* Working Paper 71. Heidelberg: Centre for Health Project Evaluation; 1997.

29 http://news.bbc.co.uk/1/hi/health/7140980.stm (accessed February 2008).

30 Webb S, Webb B. Professional associations. *New Statesman.* 1917; **9 (Special Supplement):** 7–19.

31 Tawney RH. *The Acquisitive Society.* New York: Harcourt Press; 1920.

32 Carr-Saunders AM. *Professions: their organization and place in society.* Oxford: Clarendon Press; 1928.

33 Freidson E. *Professional Powers: a study of the institutionalization of formal knowledge.* Chicago, IL: University of Chicago Press; 1986.

34 Davies S. *Against the Professions.* London: Libertarian Alliance; 1983.

35 Cruess SR, Cruess RL. Professionalism must be taught. *BMJ.* 1997; **315:** 1674–7.

36 Downie RS, Macnaughton J. *Clinical Judgment: evidence in practice.* Oxford: Oxford University Press; 2000.

37 Klein R. The state and the profession: the politics of the double bed. *BMJ.* 1990; **308:** 700–2.

38 Cruess SR, Cruess RL, Ginsburg S *et al. Evaluating Professionalism.* Workshop at the Tenth Ottawa Conference, July 2002, Ottawa, Canada.

39 Kultgen J. *Ethics and Professionalism.* Philadelphia, PA: University of Pennsylvania Press; 1988.

40 Jewson N. The disappearance of the sick man from medical cosmology, 1770–1870. *Sociology.* 1976; **10:** 225–44.

41 Porter R. *The Greatest Benefit to Mankind. A medical history of humanity from antiquity to the present.* London: Harper Collins; 1997.

42 Mishler EG. Viewpoint: critical perspectives on the biomedical model. In: Mishler EG, Amarasingham LR, Hauser ST *et al.*, editors. *Social Contexts of Health, Illness and Patient Care.* Cambridge: Cambridge University Press; 1981.

43 Percival T. *A Handbook of Medical Ethics.* London: Johnson and Bickerstaff; 1803.

44 Department of Health. *The Expert Patient: a new approach to chronic disease management for the twenty-first century.* London: The Stationery Office; 2001.

45 Shaw J, Baker M. 'Expert patient' – dream or nightmare? *BMJ.* 2004; **328:** 723–4.

46 Stevens RA. Themes in the history of medical professionalism. *Mt Sinai J Med.* 2002; **69:** 357–61.

CHAPTER 3

The code of conduct: professionalism, law and ethics

This chapter explores:
- good medical practice
- ethical duties
- ethical behaviour and ethical decision making
- legal duties
- duty of care and Good Samaritans
- medical negligence and medical malpractice
- professional advice.

> Individualism, united with altruism, has become the basis of our Western civilisation. It is the central doctrine of Christianity ('Love thy neighbour', say the Scriptures, not 'Love your tribe'); and it is the core of all ethical doctrines which have grown from our civilisations and stimulated it.
>
> *Karl Popper, 1962*[1]

One of the distinguishing features of a profession is the code of conduct to which its members agree to adhere. Often this code has been implied rather than written down. Doctors on graduation do not swear or 'profess' to uphold such a code, although many lay people believe that doctors still take the Hippocratic Oath. Certainly during most of the twentieth century, medical students learned the 'code' from the example of their tutors and doctors with whom they interacted in clinical settings. Gradually medical schools introduced courses in ethics, often as part of personal and professional development modules. Some schools also teach aspects of medical law. In the UK, the General Medical Council has set as one objective of undergraduate medical education that students should acquire a knowledge and understanding of 'ethical and legal issues relevant to the practice of medicine.'[2] Furthermore, students should demonstrate certain attitudes, including an 'awareness of the moral and ethical responsibilities involved in individual patient care and in the provision of care to populations of patients.'[2]

Since its publication in 2001, the GMC's handbook *Good Medical Practice*[3] has been used as a blueprint for the professional conduct of qualified doctors. In this respect conduct includes all features of doctor–patient and doctor–societal interactions, not specifically those that have only legal or ethical implications. Some may suggest that a code of conduct should stipulate how a doctor dresses and behaves in public, even when not officially 'on duty', whereas others might argue that such behaviour is not affecting patient care and therefore should be of no concern.

PROFESSIONAL VERSUS PRIVATE CODES OF CONDUCT

A doctor's own personal code needs to be considered. This may not be in total agreement with the code agreed by the majority of the profession. For example, there are some doctors who do not think that abortion is acceptable, and others who think that euthanasia is. This chapter concentrates on the legal and the ethical components of the code of conduct. A list of common topics included within this area is shown in Box 3.1, together with potential areas of disagreement.

BOX 3.1 LEGAL AND ETHICAL ISSUES

General issues	Areas of potential conflict
Patient autonomy	'Wants' versus 'needs' of patients; consumerism, collective versus individual decision; Western perspective
Consent to treatment	Minors; competence; Mental Health Act; benevolent paternalism
Confidentiality	Public good versus individual right to silence
Duty of care	To whom does one's duty extend?
Medical negligence	Who decides? Is it the courts, the profession or the patient?
Medical research	Ethical issues such as consent; conflicts of interest; negative findings

Doctor–patient intimacy	Misuse of power differential in relationship
Specific topics	*Areas of potential conflict*
Abortion	Not legal in all countries; may be against doctor's own beliefs; only legal in certain circumstances: who decides?
Assisted conception	Religious qualms; use of embryos; age limit; rationing – who decides?
Under-age treatment and prescribing	Moral objections to contraception; Gillick competence[4]
Mental health issues	Mental Health Act; suspension of liberties; stigmatising diagnosis
Euthanasia/assisted suicide	Illegal in the UK but not in all countries; may not be against doctor's own viewpoint; takes place illicitly
Transplantation	Opt in or opt out for donors?
Treating oneself/one's family	Is this an ethical or professional issue? Drug abuse
Female circumcision	Illegal in the UK, but cultural and religious issues need to be addressed
Torture and capital punishment	Doctors expected to be involved in certain countries

ETHICAL, LEGAL AND PROFESSIONAL DUTIES

There is a distinction between ethical practice and legal practice. There is often a difference of opinion with regard to the ethics of particular courses of action – what is 'right' and what is 'wrong' – but once a law is passed it is usually obvious what is legal and what is illegal. When doctors disagree over the ethics of a situation, or patients and their families disagree with doctors, the courts and thus the law may be invoked to pass an impartial judgment on the 'best' course of action. However, many of the ethical duties of doctors are not directly enforceable, unlike their legal duties. Doctors who fail to meet the legal standard of reasonable care in treating patients may be sued by the patients or their relatives for negligence, and may be ordered to pay compensation. Doctors who break a criminal law may be tried and convicted. Such behaviour also means that these doctors will be found guilty of professional misconduct, and may possibly have their registration and licence to practise revoked by the General Medical Council (in the UK) or other regulatory body. Breaches of the ethical code are more problematic, as these may not be liable for legal or disciplinary action.[5] In these cases, standards are often determined on the basis of what is deemed to be 'accepted practice' or what the majority of other doctors do – their code of conduct.

ETHICS IN MEDICINE

Ethics is the philosophical study of moral values and rules that govern a person's actions. We should expect professional behaviour to be equated with ethical behaviour, but the English language throws up some challenges to this relationship. For example, a *professional foul* is a term used in sport (mainly football) to define a deliberate foul committed in order to deny an opponent an advantageous position.[6] There was a mixture of outrage and admiration when the England football captain David Beckham admitted a 'professional foul' in an international match in 2004. Some of his colleagues justified his actions as 'professionalism', whereas the media tended to view them as cheating.[7]

Doctors may face dilemmas in their ethical duties, in particular when their duty to an individual patient conflicts with their duty to other patients or society as a whole. Such scenarios are often debated and the rights and wrongs argued – for example, the case of a man who tests positive for HIV and refuses to tell his wife, or the patient with epilepsy who is seen driving around town.

A fundamental ethical question is whether there is such a thing as absolute right and wrong. And stemming from this is the question of whether there is always a right way of doing things and a wrong way. Does the end always justify the means? Those who espouse the theory of consequentialism feel that the rightness of a course of action should be judged by its consequences.[8] However, this view does not sit well with the idea of a professional code of conduct, which defines action as well as outcomes. For example, I may be having a bad day and I give two patients the wrong injections. The first patient suffers no ill effects, and the second patient dies. In both cases the course of action was the same, although the drugs may have differed. The consequences were tragically different. I could make matters worse by covering up the first mistake, but it would be difficult to cover up the second one. It is obvious that my actions are wrong regardless of the outcome. Consequentialism is also open to question when the outcome is likely to be positive. If the government introduces legislation to make it impossible for a child to start school without being immunised, the herd immunity of the population is likely to increase and the number of childhood infections is likely to fall – a good outcome. However, some parents make informed choices not to have their children immunised, and they would feel coerced into a course of action about which they were unhappy. Thus, when we think of consequences, we have to ask 'the consequences for whom?' and 'who are the right people to judge?' A parent may consider that they are justified in feeling that a doctor's code of conduct should not include such coercion, but rather respect for the individual's wishes.

We may define our code according to the principle of utilitarianism, as promulgated by the liberal free thinker Jeremy Bentham (1748–1832). The concept is consequentialist. Ethical principles should produce the greatest happiness for the greatest number of people, with happiness being defined in terms of the pursuit of pleasure and the avoidance of pain.[4] This hedonistic version of life does not fit well with healthcare as such, as doctors are not primarily concerned with making patients happy, although they obviously do want to reduce physical and mental pain. Democratic governments wrestle with the problem of balancing an individual's rights with the needs of the population. Mandatory immunisation would go against some parents' right to choose, but should in theory improve the health (and therefore the happiness) of the majority of the public.

Having a code that is consequentialist does help with some of the dilemmas of practice. A man who is HIV-positive could not expect confidentiality from his doctor, given that the consequences of his continuing to practise unsafe sex would be detrimental to his partners. Thus confidentiality is not an absolute right of patients according to this concept. Indeed it is hard to think of any absolute right in healthcare that has not at some time been overridden on the basis of someone, often a doctor, deciding that the ends justify the means. However, such decisions should not be left to one person. Indeed many would say that they should not be left solely to the profession to decide. There will often be a conflict of interest. This is why lay people need to be involved in deciding what is acceptable behaviour for doctors.

THE DUTIES OF A DOCTOR

In contrast to consequentialism, the philosopher Immanuel Kant (1724–1804) wrote of duty and the importance of what a person is thinking when choices are being made. We should not act out of self-interest, or because such an action makes us feel good, or because of what we hope to be the consequences of our actions, but out of duty, and respect for the moral law. Kant defined moral law in terms of the categorical imperative – that is, we should act only according to those principles that we would want to be a universal law. In other words, would you want to live in a world in which everyone was acting in the same way that you propose to act?[9]

Deontologists – people who act through a sense of duty (from *deon*, the Greek word for duty) – believe that morals may be defined, that they are independent of the consequences of an action, and that there are thus absolute rights and wrongs. The problem that the deontologists face is how we know what is right and what is wrong. For some the answer is simple. God decides, and religion interprets these decisions. For others, rights and wrongs are defined by society, but societies evolve or mature and rights and wrongs need to be constantly reinterpreted. For example, abortion is now legal in some countries where once it was illegal. The government, acting to some extent on society's wishes, has defined 'right' as applied to a woman's right to choose. However, the followers of many religions would still define abortion as morally wrong. When, therefore, should doctors update their professional codes, especially if they conflict with their personal codes of conduct?

BOX 3.2 THE DUTIES OF A DOCTOR[11]

As a doctor you must:

- make the care of your patient your first concern
- treat every patient politely and considerately
- respect patients' dignity and privacy
- listen to patients and respect their views
- give patients information in a way that they can understand
- respect the rights of patients to be fully involved in decisions about their care
- keep your professional knowledge and skills up to date
- recognise the limits of your professional competence
- be honest and trustworthy
- respect and protect confidential information
- make sure that your personal beliefs do not prejudice your patients' care
- act quickly to protect patients from risk if you have good reason to believe that you or a colleague may not be fit to practise
- avoid abusing your position as a doctor
- work with colleagues in the ways that best serve patients' interests.

In all these matters you must never discriminate unfairly against your patients or colleagues. And you must always be prepared to justify your actions to them.

Duties to others are defined by our relationships. Doctors have obligations to their patients that they do not have to other people with whom they interact.[10] In the UK, the duties of a doctor have been defined by the General Medical Council (*see* Box 3.2).[11]

Few people would argue with any of the duties listed in Box 3.2. They are fairly broad, and avoid mentioning specifically the more contentious ethical issues such as abortion and sectioning of patients under the Mental Health Act. However, on further reflection, some of them are open to interpretation and do require further definition.

Although in most circumstances doctors do make the care of patients their first concern, many doctors will remember instances where this was not the case. Usually this involves making a judgement about the urgency of a patient's needs. For instance, if a general practitioner is seeing the last patient of the day, is already running an hour behind schedule, and another patient contacts the surgery and asks to be seen for a problem that is (to the doctor) seemingly trivial, it is unlikely that the doctor will see the patient that night.

Should we respect all the views of our patients? What if a patient makes a racist remark about a doctor and refuses to be referred to certain doctors because of their race? An article published in the *British Medical Journal* in 1999 gave a variety of answers to the questions of how doctors should behave with a racist patient. These included telling the patient that they disagree with their views without bullying, isolation of the patient from others, and withdrawal of treatment.[12] We may also respect a patient's views without necessarily acting upon them. Sometimes it may be impossible to do so, because the patient's desired course of action is illegal (e.g. assisted suicide). Involving the patient in and then respecting a decision on management may also cause problems. Although we may feel uncomfortable if a patient chooses not to follow advice on treatment after receiving all of the necessary information, we respect the patient's decision. For example, a patient may decline to take tablets to lower their cholesterol level, or a Jehovah's Witness may decline a blood transfusion. However, we do not usually respect a patient's decision to do something that we think is medically unsound or unproven. For example, a 36-year-old woman who smokes 30 cigarettes a day and who wishes to carry on taking the combined oral contraceptive pill despite the risks is unlikely to find a doctor who is willing to prescribe it.

Working in ways that best serve patients' interests is difficult, because of the problem of who decides on what is their best interest. Should it be the doctor concerned, other doctors, the patient, or the family? (Further discussion of professional and patient autonomy can be found in Chapter 9.)

DECIDING ON AN ETHICAL CODE

Moral pluralism is a feature of modern society. There is often not one moral solution to a problem. Our culturally diverse population means that there are many secular and religious viewpoints. Doctors and other health professionals reflect this multiculturalism and have different ideas as to what is the correct course of action in some ethically problematic clinical situations. However, medical students should be trained to be able to think and to argue and critique the behaviour of their tutors and those who act as role models. Subsequently, doctors will be able to deliberate ethically by drawing on their theoretical knowledge and their experience. So while there may not be one absolutely correct moral choice, there may be one option that is 'better, more rigorous and inclusive than others.'[11] Doctors should also revisit ethics during their continuing professional development, and be able to challenge one another's assumptions and reflect on their experiences.

BOX 3.3 THE FOUR PRINCIPLES OF ETHICAL BEHAVIOUR[13]

Justice: concepts of fairness, rightness and equity.
Autonomy: includes self-determination, liberty, rights and free will.
Non-maleficence: to do no harm.
Beneficence: active well doing, altruism.

BOX 3.4 A MODEL OF ETHICAL DECISION MAKING[8]

- Clearly state the problem (definition).
- Identify the facts (listen to the patient, carers, and health professionals involved).
- Consider the four ethical principles and how they impact on the problem.
- Consider how the problem would look from another perspective (e.g. feminist, lay person, consequentialist, religious).
- Identify ethical conflicts.
- Consider legal aspects.
- Make the ethical decision (and evaluate it).

Kerridge *et al.*[8] have developed a model for ethical decision making which incorporates the four fundamental ethical principles of Beauchamp and Childress[13] (*see* Box 3.3). In the latter part of the twentieth century, the principle of individual patient autonomy was paramount. However, a shift is now occurring towards a greater concentration on justice, in recognition of the fact that the healthcare choices of the poorer nations are constrained by inequality in resources. The decision-making model may be applied in clinical situations to decide on the best course of action (*see* Box 3.4).

'IT IS MY RIGHT'

Patients have rights, although they are not always clear what those rights are. When considering the definition of what a right is, some claims become obviously ridiculous. A right is a justifiable claim that an individual or group can make upon society or other individuals. A decade ago many people believed that they had the right to a home visit. 'I know my rights, doctor.' Patients' rights are related to doctors' duties. Society or individuals have duties to uphold people's rights. A patient has the right to expect that a doctor will do his or her duty. However, even here the issue is not completely clear. Does the person have to be a *patient* of this particular doctor? And what makes a doctor–patient relationship in this context? If the patient is registered with the doctor and has a consultation with the doctor, then the patient has a right to appropriate care. GPs in the UK are also required to give 'immediately necessary' care to non-registered patients under certain circumstances – for example, in the event of accidents and in emergencies. With regard to secondary and tertiary care, once the hospital staff have accepted a patient for treatment, they owe a duty of care. If the person has a medical problem and asks for help or advice from a doctor in a social situation, does the same duty apply? In other words, does a doctor's code of conduct apply 24 hours a day and/or can a doctor ever be really 'off duty'?

The concept of rights dates back to the English Bill of Rights that was passed in 1689. This was an act declaring the rights and liberties of the subject and settling the succession of the crown, following the 'Glorious Revolution' when James II fled the country and William and Mary of Orange succeeded to the throne.[14] These rights refer to individuals being free from the arbitrary interference of the state, and include the right to freedom of speech, religious freedom, assembly and the right to due process under the law of the land.

In 1994, the United Nations issued an 'International Covenant on Economic, Social and Cultural Rights.'[15] Article 12 is shown in Box 3.5. These rights were not recognised in full by all countries, but could reasonably be expected to form part of a doctor's code of conduct at a personal and population level.

BOX 3.5 ARTICLE 12 OF THE INTERNATIONAL COVENANT[15]

1 The States Parties to the present Covenant recognise the right of everyone to the enjoyment of the highest attainable standard of physical and mental health.
2 The steps to be taken by the States Parties to the present Covenant to achieve the full realisation of this right shall include those necessary for:
  - the provision for the reduction of the stillbirth rate and of infant mortality and for the healthy development of the child
  - the improvement of all aspects of environmental and industrial hygiene
  - the prevention, treatment and control of epidemic, endemic, occupational and other diseases
  - the creation of conditions that would assure to all medical service and medical attention in the event of sickness.

The legal duties of a doctor are listed in Box 3.6.[4] These translate into patients' rights. The first, of course, still requires definition. Many of them are similar to the duties of a doctor listed above, but the legal aspect indicates that doctors may be sued or judged to have acted illegally if they breach any of them.

BOX 3.6 LEGAL DUTIES OF A DOCTOR

- Meet professional standards.
- Take reasonable care.
- Provide information to patients.
- Maintain confidentiality.
- Do not treat or detain patients without consent unless there is legal justification.
- Follow up patients.
- Preserve life.
- Do not perform unlawful abortions.
- Report notifiable diseases.
- Report deaths.
- Report child abuse.
- Report drug abusers.
- Write true and accurate records/certificates.
- Act in the patient's best interests.

THE GOOD SAMARITAN

The difference between the moral duty and the legal duty of a doctor may be illustrated by the concept of the 'Good Samaritan'. In healthcare this refers to a health professional assisting in an emergency when not officially 'on duty'. In the UK, doctors have no legal obligation to help the injured in such cases,[7] although many would regard it as their moral duty. The GMC has issued the guidance that 'In an emergency, wherever it may arise, you must offer anyone at risk the assistance you could reasonably be expected to provide',[10] reinforcing the moral obligation. This is the same for any lay person, who would not be expected to leave an injured or sick human being unaided. The standard of care offered would of course be different. It is possible for a doctor to be sued in such circumstances if the standard of care applied is suboptimal, although such outcomes are rare. Thus everyone has a moral duty to help another. This has been interpreted as showing that for doctors there is nothing special about their obligation. They have no special moral duties compared with the rest of the population.[16] Only their legal duties are different because of their profession.

FIRST, DO NO HARM

Although this phrase is often quoted in the Latin *primum non nocere*, it appears to originate from the Greek of Hippocrates, who wrote 'As to diseases, make a habit of two things – to help, or at least to do no harm.'[17] Should non-maleficence have a higher standing in the doctor's code than beneficence? Worry about causing harm may indeed prevent a doctor from trying to help a patient. Such considerations are important for informed consent, when patients are given information not only about the possible benefits of a procedure or treatment, but also about the adverse events that might occur. Such discussion of risk is a difficult undertaking for many doctors and their patients, both of whom may have little understanding of how risk should be communicated. Patients are influenced by a number of factors when listening to information about risk, one of which is the extent to which they trust the person (the doctor) who is talking to them.[18]

Doctors also withhold information from patients due to a fear of causing harm. In the past, doctors – acting paternalistically – have tried to shield their patients from poor prognoses, even considering it inhumane or detrimental to them to be honest about their diagnoses.[19] Even today this may happen at the request of family members who are reluctant to have bad news broken to their relative 'in case he cannot cope'. Although all concerned are acting in what they consider to be the best interests of the patient, we need to consider how we determine what those best interests are. Surely it is up to the patient to define his or her own best interests if at all possible. Of course there are numerous examples of situations where this is not possible or allowable. For example, if the patient is a child, or is mentally unwell or unconscious, someone else is given the power to make a decision.

PATIENT SAFETY

The exhortation to 'do no harm' as a personal mantra for the caring doctor is ironic when viewed against the figures relating to medical errors and adverse effects within healthcare services. The Department of Health's publication of 2000, *An Organisation with a Memory*, reviews the causes and effects of medical error and lists some estimated annual statistics relating to this (*see* Box 3.7).[20] Around 10% of hospital admissions result in iatrogenic harm to patients.

BOX 3.7 FIGURES RELATING TO PATIENT SAFETY[20]
(ESTIMATED ANNUAL NUMBER)

Written complaints regarding care and treatment in hospitals	27 949
Written complaints regarding care and treatment in primary care	38 857
Serious untoward events/incidents	2 500
Adverse events (including 87 deaths)	6 610
Adverse drug reactions	18 196

The patient safety issue is of great concern to the NHS. Errors often arise from imperfect systems rather than individual forgetfulness, incompetence or malice[21] (*see also* Chapter 9). However, doctors have been slow to embrace the fact that this is the case,[22] while patients tend to blame a specific single doctor for serious mistakes.[23]

One might expect that a doctor's ethical code would involve being open and honest about mistakes. Such honesty would be easier in a system that did not punish individuals. However, human nature often leads to covering up, deflecting blame or lying about incidents, especially as a doctor's livelihood and reputation are at stake. The dishonest doctor transgresses both ethical and legal codes, as covering up often means altering notes, which is fraudulent, so can hardly be described as professional behaviour.

MEDICAL MALPRACTICE

Medical malpractice is defined as 'any unjustified act or failure to act upon the part of a doctor or other healthcare worker which results in harm to the patient.'[7] The majority of malpractice claims by patients are made in relation to alleged negligence by a doctor. Patients may also sue because of battery, but this is rare. Battery occurs when examination or treatment is carried out without consent (i.e. there is non-consensual touching). For assault to occur, a person must be aware of an impending threat. This is of course not possible when a patient is anaesthetised.

A common scenario relating to battery is the conducting of physical examinations by medical students on patients who are asleep. The Royal College of Obstetricians and Gynaecologists[24] and the Department of Health[25] have issued guidelines relating to medical training and intimate examinations (usually rectal and vaginal examinations). However, a study carried out in 2003 suggested that, in many teaching hospitals, students were either performing such examinations without consent or they did not know whether consent had been given.[26] Perhaps the doctors concerned did not consider the ethics of the situation; they certainly did not appear to know that they were breaking the law.

Clinical negligence is defined, somewhat inelegantly, by the Department of Health as 'A breach of duty of care by members of the healthcare professions employed by NHS bodies or by others consequent on decisions or judgements made by members of those professions acting in their professional capacity in the course of their employment, and which are admitted as negligent by the employer or are determined as such through the legal processes.'[27] Negligence results in harm to patients, and such patients or their relatives may sue for damages in court.

Of course any person may make a mistake. It is a professional duty to minimise the risks of such a possibility by keeping up to date, paying adequate attention to one's health, including one's physical and psychological well-being, seeking help when necessary and, importantly, recognising one's own limitations within a given clinical situation. Negligence claims hinge on the prosecution being able to show that the health professional concerned had a duty of care to the patient, that the negligent action contributed to the patient's harm, and that the defendant did not behave in a manner consistent with accepted medical opinion or standard care.

The latter condition is often difficult to prove. The famous case that is used as the benchmark for such decisions is *Bolam v Friern Hospital Management Committee* of 1957,[28] which resulted in the establishment of the *Bolam test* or *Bolam principle*. The test states that a doctor is not negligent if he or she acts in accordance with what is accepted as proper by a responsible body of his or her own peers. These peers will be at the same level of training and expertise. Lord Scarman, in the case of *Sidaway v Governors of Bethlem Royal Hospital* in 1985, made the infamous remark that 'The law imposes the duty of care: but the standard of care is a matter of medical judgement.'[29] This leaves the profession with a great deal of leeway and the potential for 'closing ranks', to the detriment of patients. Moreover, there is a problem in that, even in these days of evidence-based practice, not all specialists within a particular field agree on what is an optimum management plan. Medical witnesses are employed by lawyers to state what, in their opinion, is an acceptable standard of care. Counsel then has to prove that these witnesses are indeed experts; the court makes a judgement on this expertise rather than on what the experts are actually saying. In other words, courts do not decide on what is technical competence. Some legal commentators feel that this is an excessively deferential attitude towards medical opinion, but believe that it arose in order to deter an explosion of medical negligence cases and to preserve trust between doctors and patients[6]. However, more recently, courts have been encouraged to evaluate the medical evidence, even when medical experts give it. In the case of *Bolitho v City and Hackney HA* in 1997, Lord Browne-Wilkinson stated that the court must examine the logical basis of the expert opinion and in particular consider the comparative risks and benefits of any treatment under consideration.[30] However, he also expressed the opinion that it would be rare for a court to substitute its own judgement for that of the experts.[30]

WHERE TO FIND HELP

Doctors who require help with legal or ethical issues have a number of options when seeking advice. Their defence organisations are useful sources of support and information. Colleagues, local ethical committees and the GMC may also help.

SUMMARY

Professionalism involves professionals having a code of conduct. However, who defines this code, what its boundaries are, and whether professionals agree with one another about the items are all issues that need discussion. Various bodies have suggested codes which may incorporate ethical and/or legal responsibilities. Codes vary between countries and over time. Nationally imposed codes may not be compatible with personal morals.

REFERENCES

1 Popper KR. *Open Society and Its Enemies. Volume 1. Plato.* Princeton, NJ: Princeton Paperback Printing; 1971.
2 General Medical Council. *Tomorrow's Doctors.* London: General Medical Council; 1993.
3 General Medical Council. *Good Medical Practice.* London: General Medical Council; 2001.
4 Stauch M, Wheat K, Tingle J. *Sourcebook on Medical Law.* 2nd ed. London: Cavendish Publishing Limited; 2002.
5 Skene L. *Law and Medical Practice: rights, duties, claims and defences.* Sydney: Butterworths; 1998.
6 Oxford University Press. *Oxford Dictionary of English.* 2nd ed. Oxford: Oxford University Press; 2003.
7 Professional foul. *The Guardian,* 13 October 2004.
8 Kerridge I, Lowe M, McPhee J. *Ethics and Law for the Health Professions.* 2nd ed. Sydney: The Federation Press; 2005.
9 Kant I (Gregor MJ, Sullivan RJ, editors). *The Fundamental Principles of the Metaphysics of Morals.* Cambridge: Cambridge University Press; 1996 (originally published 1785).
10 Beauchamp TL, Walters L. *Contemporary Issues in Bioethics.* Belmont, CA: Wadsworth Publishing; 1982.
11 General Medical Council. *The Duties of a Doctor.* London: General Medical Council; 2002.
12 Beauchamp TL, Childress J. *Principles of Biomedical Ethics.* New York: Oxford University Press; 2001.
13 Selby M, Neuberger J, Easmon C et al. Ethical dilemma: dealing with racist patients. *BMJ.* 1999; **318:** 1129–31.
14 www.fordham.edu/halsall/mod/1689billofrights.html (accessed May 2008).
15 www.hrweb.org/legal/escr.html (accessed May 2008).
16 Harris J. *The Value of Life.* London: Routledge and Kegan Paul; 1985.
17 Hippocrates. *Epidemics* (Smith WD, trans.). Boston, MA: Loeb Classical Library; 1994.
18 Alaszewski A, Horlick-Jones T. How can doctors communicate information about risk more effectively? *BMJ.* 2003; **327:** 695–6.
19 Oken D. What to tell cancer patients: a study of medical attitudes. *JAMA.* 1961; **175:** 1120–28.
20 Department of Health. *An Organisation with a Memory.* London: The Stationery Office; 2000.
21 Reason J. Human error: models and management. *BMJ.* 2000; **320:** 768–70.
22 Stryer D, Clancy C. Patients' safety. *BMJ.* 2005; **330:** 553–4.
23 Blendon RJ, DesRoches CM, Brodie M et al. Views of practicing physicians and the public on medical errors. *NEJM.* 2002; **347:** 1933–40.
24 Royal College of Obstetricians and Gynaecologists. *Intimate Examinations: Report of a Working Party.* London: RCOG Press; 1997.
25 Department of Health. *Reference Guide to Consent for Examination and Treatment.* London: The Stationery Office; 2001.
26 Coldicott Y, Pope C, Roberts C. The ethics of intimate examinations – teaching tomorrow's doctors. *BMJ.* 2003; **326:** 97–101.

27 Department of Health. *NHS Indemnity: arrangements for negligence claims in the NHS.* London: The Stationery Office; 1996.

28 *Bolam v Friern Hospital Management Committee* [1957] 1 WLR 582.

29 *Sidaway v Governors of Bethlem Royal Hospital and the Maudsley Hospital* [1985] 1 All ER 1018, HL.

30 *Bolitho v City and Hackney HA* [1997] 4 All ER 771, HL.

CHAPTER 4

Professional–patient relationships

This chapter explores:
- the nature of the professional–patient relationship
- sexual intimacy and professionalism
- the case for chaperones
- dealing with aggression
- boundary violations
- presents from patients
- presents from drug companies – doctors and the drug industry
- the nature of empathy.

> Somewhere in our more primitive depths is a lust, half childish, half sadistic, to use whatever power we might have to victimize others, and enjoy it – to glory in the fact that they and not we are the victims, and to escape for a moment into the fantasy that since we can avoid the victimhood through our power, we are invulnerable and need never again feel fear.
>
> *H Brody, The Healer's Power, 1992*[1]

If we were to ask members of the public what bad behaviour would automatically lead to a doctor being 'struck off' the medical register, many would probably answer 'having sex with a patient.' Inappropriate relationships with patients are a well-known taboo. We now also talk about boundary issues and 'professional' relationships. There is a lot more to what constitutes a professional relationship than the absence of overt sexual intimacy. In contrast to many other aspects of professionalism, perhaps many health professionals would say that avoiding sex with patients/clients is easy. However, the demise of the paternalistic doctor–patient relationship of the nineteenth and twentieth centuries has raised some interesting questions about equality, partnership and what exactly is the nature of the professional–patient bond. One of the recurring themes of professional–patient relationships is power.

(The themes of this chapter are also taken up later in this book with different emphases – on shared decision making in Chapter 5, and consumerism in Chapter 9.)

DOCTOR–PATIENT SEXUAL RELATIONSHIPS

The Hippocratic Oath (*see* Chapter 2) includes the following lines: 'Whatever houses I may visit, I will come for the benefit of the sick, remaining free of all intentional injustice, of all mischief and in particular of sexual relations with both female and male persons, be they free or slaves.'[2] In the context of ancient Greek civilisation, this part of the oath may be seen as protecting a doctor's reputation, income and the prestige of his calling, rather than serving as a safeguard for the welfare of patients under his care.[3]

Within many societies, doctors have an unusual degree of freedom with regard to intimacy that is not often granted to non-family members – hence the need for a code of conduct from the earliest times to define the limits of this intimacy. Doctor–patient consultations should take place in a neutral environment of trust and confidentiality. However, a neutral environment is difficult to define. The doctor's office seems to belong to the doctor, is familiar to the doctor, but is often strange and perhaps frightening to the patient. A consulting room should be clinical (a place where medical practice takes place) and of a fairly standard specification. Yet it should also be welcoming and ease the patient's disclosure of what may be embarrassing and personal details. The home visit is potentially fraught with danger. The possible scenario of a scantily dressed female patient lying in bed in an otherwise empty house is a good reason for insisting that intimate examinations are carried out in the surgery and not in the patient's home.

The doctor's white coat and the nurse's uniform – the badge of their professional personas – in some ways act as barriers to personal relationships. However, in many clinical situations doctors no longer wear a white coat, in order to help to break down these barriers – for example, in psychiatry and paediatrics. The nurse's heavily starched apron and hat of bygone eras are no longer worn. Instead, nurses wear more comfortable and practical apparel that perhaps makes them appear less official. In most cases, doctors no longer sit behind a desk with the patient on the opposite side, but rather patient and doctor interact across the corner of the desk, closer together. But now we have the distraction of the computer on the desk instead, and it is perhaps a more intrusive object than a chunk of wood. Health professionals are nearer their patients in some ways, but more distant in others.

Even without considering intimate examinations, in past centuries male doctors were able to look upon parts of the female anatomy – ankles, knees, chest and abdomen – that were forbidden to the rest of male society. Even for the most embarrassed woman there was an element of safety and trust because this man to whom her body was exposed was a professional, a doctor and a highly regarded member of society. The power differential in such relationships is easy to see. Not only was there the prevailing power imbalance between male and female, but also here between learned and ignorant.

The General Medical Council stipulates that 'you must not allow your personal relationships to undermine the trust which patients place in you. In particular you must not use your professional position to establish or pursue a sexual or improper emotional relationship with a patient or someone close to them.'[4] In 2006, the GMC issued new guidance focusing on the feeling that the relationship between a patient and a doctor is never really equal. Its previous guidance was only concerned with intimacy between doctors and current patients, but this more recent document extends the caution to former patients. Although it does not recommend a complete ban on sexual relationships, and indeed recognises that there are always exceptions to the rules, the GMC with this document aims to protect vulnerable patients.[5] The 1983 and older version of the rules for professional conduct highlight the fact that doctors may have received confidential information about the state of a patient's marriage that may lead them into professional misconduct.[6]

Ian Kerridge and colleagues quote some statistics in their book on medical ethics and law relating to the prevalence of sexual behaviour between health professionals and patients in the USA. The figures are over 10 years old, but still make interesting reading. Sexual feelings for patients are common, with 95% of male psychologists and 75% of female psychologists reporting such feelings at least once in their careers. Figures for actual sexual relationships are more difficult to find, but Kerridge quoted a figure of 5–10% of psychiatrists having had sex with patients.[7] Most of the available statistics relating to sexual relationships concern psychiatrists more than any other medical specialty. However, health professionals are not unique in transgressing acceptable professional behaviour. Teachers and priests are the subjects of many complaints to their relevant authorities. Because of the power imbalance inherent in such relationships and the possible long-term adverse consequences for patients, these situations have been likened to rape and incest.[8] Patients may develop problems such as depression, anxiety disorders, psychosexual dysfunction, inability to trust health professionals in future encounters, guilt and feelings of worthlessness, and increased drug and alcohol use. The types of behaviour that would constitute sexual misconduct are listed in Box 4.1. Although in most cases health professionals enter into a sexual relationship with one patient only, a small number of health professionals act in a predatory way and prey on a succession of patients.

BOX 4.1 EXAMPLES OF SEXUAL MISCONDUCT

- Conducting intimate examinations without permission (e.g. while the patient is anaesthetised or unconscious).
- Rendering the patient in such a state that they were unable to refuse intimacy (e.g. giving the patient drugs, hypnotising the patient).
- Rape.
- Conducting an unnecessary physical examination, such as pelvic or breast examination.
- Frotteurism (achieving sexual stimulation or orgasm by touching and rubbing against a patient).
- Watching the patient undressing.
- Using overt sexual language that is unnecessary in that consultation.

The other aspect of this topic that needs to be considered concerns doctors in sexual relationships with people who later become patients – for example, a doctor who wishes to treat his or her spouse or same-sex partner. This may be considered necessary if the family lives in a remote area where there is no other medical help available. The guidelines against treating family members are discussed in Chapter 8.

WHAT ABOUT FORMER PATIENTS?

As mentioned above, the GMC now warns against sexual relationships with former patients.[5] Twenty years ago, an American survey found that nearly 30% of psychiatrists thought that having sex with a patient after termination of counselling was not inappropriate.[9] Katherine Hall of the Department of General Practice, University of Otago, New Zealand, believes that sexual relationships with former patients should not be regarded as ethically permissible except under rare circumstances.[10] Her argument is again based on the power differential between the two individuals. The Medical Council of New Zealand has produced two booklets, *The Importance of Clear Sexual Boundaries in the*

Doctor–Patient Relationship 2004 (a guide for patients) and *Sexual Boundaries in the Doctor–Patient Relationship 2004* (a guide for doctors).[11] These policy documents in particular highlight that the Council will consider it to be unethical if the doctor–patient relationship prior to sexual intimacy involved counselling or psychotherapy. The Council also warns against sexual relationships with former patients suffering from medical conditions that are likely to affect their decision making and/or impair their judgement, patients with a history of sexual abuse, and patients under the age of 20 years when the doctor–patient relationship ended. In the guide for patients, patients are advised of their own responsibilities to tell the doctor to stop if he or she is doing something that makes the patient feel uncomfortable, or if the patient wants to ask questions about what is happening. However, many patients would probably not feel able to do this because of their perceptions of the doctor's power compared with their own feelings of vulnerability.

CHAPERONES AND INTIMATE EXAMINATIONS

In modern times, in societies where men and women expose much more of their bodies in public than has been the custom for many generations, the risk of impropriety, paradoxically, is regarded as more likely. Hence the recommendation that doctors and other health professionals who are performing intimate (and even non-intimate) examinations should have a chaperone. This safety measure is also seen as protecting doctors as well as patients. This shows how times have changed, as doctors feel themselves to be at risk of false accusations of sexual harassment or even physical and sexual assault. The NHS Clinical Governance Support Team has published a model chaperone framework. It states that 'for most patients respect, explanation, consent and privacy take precedence over the need for a chaperone. The presence of a third party does not negate the need for adequate explanation and courtesy and cannot provide full assurance that the procedure or examination is conducted appropriately.'[12] The Royal College of Obstetricians and Gynaecologists recommends that patients who need to undergo intimate examinations should be offered a chaperone irrespective of the gender of the doctor or nurse who is performing the physical examination, and that if the patient declines, this request should be honoured and noted in the medical records.[13] Since the 1980s and 1990s the use of chaperones by male doctors has increased substantially, but chaperone use by female doctors is still low, and record keeping about offers and the presence or absence of a chaperone is still poor.[14]

Surveys have shown that most women would like to be offered a chaperone, but feel uncomfortable asking for one if the offer is not made. This is more likely to be the case if the doctor is male, and a female nurse is then usually the third party of choice.[15] In the (female) author's own general practice women prefer not to have a third party present at all, even a female medical student in many cases. If a patient does want or ask for a chaperone, the excuse that no one is available is not acceptable, and the examination should be postponed until a chaperone is available. Doctors may be accused of unprofessional conduct if they do not have a chaperone present. Unprofessional conduct in this context includes overexposure of the patient's body, inappropriate comments, inappropriate gestures or body language, and putting the patient in an unorthodox position.[16]

Good communication is vital for preventing misunderstandings about the nature and purpose of physical examinations. Men who request a blood test for prostate screening would not usually expect a rectal examination to be part of the package. Similarly, women with abdominal pain and bloating may not understand the relevance of a pelvic bimanual examination without adequate explanation.

PHYSICAL AND SEXUAL HARASSMENT BY PATIENTS

Of course not all patients are innocent victims of power-hungry or misguided health professionals. Patients under the influence of drugs or alcohol, or with antisocial behavioural problems, may make sexual advances to healthcare staff, or use sexual and/or abusive language. Holding a patient's hand or giving a patient a hug may be misinterpreted by the patient as more than a therapeutic gesture. Some patients may 'fancy' their nurse or doctor – sexual attraction can and does arise in many situations. If a health professional considers that the feelings of a patient are outside the ethical relationship, the professional must discuss this with the patient and if necessary arrange for them to be treated by someone else.

A British Medical Association survey of 3000 doctors in 2003 found that violence against doctors was common, with psychiatrists and doctors working in Accident and Emergency departments being the most frequently affected.[17] Verbal abuse by patients and their relatives occurs most often, but physical assault is also common. The professional response is not to retaliate, but to take avoiding action and call for help. A brawl involving a healthcare worker and a patient or relative does nothing for the professional persona of the worker. Being alert to the signs of impending violence helps to prevent escalation of violence. Patients become angry in situations when conflict arises and their wants or demands are unmet, when they receive bad news, or during emotional and stressful interviews. Although anger is common, overt aggression is relatively rare. Patients with a history of violence or substance abuse are more likely to switch to become aggressive, and this applies to patients of any age.[18] Health professionals need to be able to deal with these situations, and this requires training. However, such training is rarely given, and lack of support following a violent incidence is common.[17]

Signs that a person is becoming angry include an increase in respiratory rate, speech becoming louder, facial flushing and obvious tension in the neck and shoulders. When a patient becomes angry, the health professional should acknowledge this and try to explore the reasons for the emotion while being careful not to invade the patient's personal space. Empathic statements (and see below) such as 'I can see that you are angry' may be helpful in defusing the situation. Simple statements of fact followed by invitations to discuss the problem may be made – for example, 'I noticed that you were very angry with the receptionist – would you like to tell me why?' Strategies for dealing with angry or aggressive patients are listed in Box 4.2.

BOX 4.2 STRATEGIES FOR DEALING WITH ANGRY PATIENTS

- If both of you are standing up, sit down yourself and then invite the patient to sit down.
- If you are seated, do not stand up, but invite the angry person to sit down.
- Move to a private area if appropriate, but ensure that your personal safety is not compromised.
- Use an appropriate tone of voice – do not shout, speak over the patient or interrupt them.
- Face the other person squarely and maintain eye contact.
- Appear confident and professional.
- Be firm as appropriate.
- Do not give in to inappropriate demands.
- Apologise if this is appropriate. Admit your mistakes.
- Allow time to de-stress after the interview. Don't rush straight on to the next patient.

MEDICAL POWER

The movement from paternalism (the practice of treating people in a fatherly manner, providing for their needs without giving them rights or responsibilities) towards patient-centred care[19] has been well documented, and has resulted in many of the changes with regard to the professional–patient relationship that have taken place over the last 20 years. Thus we have shared decision making, informed consent, patient participation groups and the *Patient's Charter*.[20]

However much we maintain that there is partnership in doctor–patient interactions, there will always be a power differential – differences in knowledge and skills, and the doctor having the right to issue or refuse a prescription or medical certificate. Even when doctors give patients choices with regard to management, they may only give certain choices, based on their own biases, availability and costs. Eliot Freidson, the American sociologist, suggested over 30 years ago that doctors deliberately withhold information from patients in order to maintain their professional dominance and power.[21] This stems from their 'splendid isolation' from society at large, and leads to the exertion of an unreasonable level of social control.[22] Things may have changed, but there is still the potential for abuse of power and inappropriate behaviour.

We may think of power in three dimensions. In the first dimension, A forces B to do something. In the second, A controls the agenda in any interaction with B. In the third dimension, A controls the world as B sees it. The third dimensional view of power is relevant to the decision-making process within a consultation.[23] B (the patient) will make a decision based on the information received from A (the doctor). Thus B's actions are shaped by the medical knowledge supplied by A. B may have a free choice of options, but only of those options that A has decided to supply. A in fact still holds the balance of power within the doctor–patient relationship. According to Brody, a family physician and ethicist, the goal is to exercise the ethical use of power by the physician on the patient's behalf.[1]

Brody defines three types of medical power – Aesculapian, charismatic and social.[1] Aesculapian power is the medical power that doctors have by virtue of training and the body of professional knowledge they possess. Charismatic power is due to the personality of the doctor and the way in which they interact with patients. Social power comes from doctors' position within society. It is the latter which is probably most under threat from the various attacks on professional status outlined in Chapter 9.

Of course patients exercise their power in refusing or declining to do what the doctor tells them. For example, they may continue to smoke, they may not take their medication as prescribed, or they may not return for their follow-up appointment. However, this is a very different power from that of the professional who, in gatekeeper health services, is able to decide on investigations, referrals and certification. Doctors may complain that patients are manipulating them into giving prescriptions for antibiotics and narcotics, or handing out certificates for that extra week off work. However, in reality doctors have almost total control of the way that the doctor–patient relationship is run, including appointment times, length of appointment, choice of venue, when to carry out procedures, giving out results of tests and investigations, and availability out of hours. Unless and until patients can exercise the right to challenge and reject the preferences of their doctor (or other health professional), they can draw no effective personal boundaries between themselves and these preferences.[24]

BOUNDARY VIOLATIONS

Health professionals and patients interact within a therapeutic relationship. Once either professional or patient begin to act in such as way as to satisfy non-therapeutic desires or goals, the behaviour is defined as a boundary violation. There is a distinction between a boundary crossing and a violation. Crossings are not exploitative and may be helpful to the patient, but violations are always harmful.[25] Sexual relationships often develop after a series of boundary crossings.[25] Such behaviour includes not only sexual intimacy but also giving and receiving information for financial rewards, giving or exchanging expensive gifts, and borrowing or lending money.

Boundary violations, particularly those of a sexual nature, often arise through the phenomena of transference and counter-transference.[7] These terms derive from the psychoanalytical school of psychiatry, but are common phenomena in many consultations over long periods of time. Transference refers to the feelings that the patient has for the therapist (the doctor or other health professional), which often mirror those that he or she has had for authority figures in the past. Such feelings may be therapeutic in that they provide insight into relationship problems in the past. The feelings for the therapist may involve affection and sexual attraction. Counter-transference refers to the feelings that the therapist (the doctor or other health professional) has for the patient. These feelings may arise due to the patient's displays of affection.

Although boundary violations may occur due to the power imbalance of the relationship, they are also likely to occur if the doctor tries to bring the interaction on to a more even level. If the professional persona of the doctor is played down by dress, attitude, informal speech or easy accessibility, the patient may feel more able to express intimate feelings. Although it has been the custom for many years for health professionals to call patients by their first name, increasingly patients are beginning to act in a similar way. Health professionals may feel that discussing their own life helps to break down barriers between them and their patient, thus enhancing the patient's own ability to disclose intimate details about their medical history and lifestyle.

However, such discussion may lead a vulnerable patient to believe that the professional–patient relationship has a life and meaning outside the consulting room. Professionals face the difficulty of adopting an empathic consulting style which may be therapeutic, but which could also enhance a more destructive transference/counter-transference relationship.

Boundary violations may also occur if a health professional tries to impose his or her own moral views on a patient – for example, if a doctor refuses to discuss contraception with a patient on religious grounds, and does not refer them to a doctor who will discuss the subject. Some doctors tell patients off for their 'bad behaviour', such as sexual relationships before marriage. Giving patients advice about risky behaviour such as unsafe sex is appropriate, but only if the doctor does not do this in a judgemental way. Telling gay patients that their life choice is sinful is certainly not appropriate. Health professionals also abuse their authority if they try to advance their own political agendas. They should think carefully about putting their name publicly to any political campaign, and they should not encourage patients to donate money to inappropriate causes by placing collection boxes in their workplaces.

BOX 4.3 WARNING – BOUNDARY VIOLATION!

- Seeking the patient's company outside the consulting room.
- Telling patients personal/intimate details about yourself.
- Telling patients your own problems.
- Accepting presents from patients.
- Giving presents to patients.
- Comparing a patient with your current sexual partner/spouse.
- Thinking that a patient's life would be better if they have sex with you.
- Feeling excited before the patient's next appointment.
- Daydreaming about the patient.
- Feeling proud that a famous person is your patient.
- Enjoying the feeling that you have power over a patient.
- Asking a patient to do personal favours for you, such as posting a letter.
- Making special arrangements for a patient, such as seeing them after surgery hours.

There are warning signs of boundaries becoming fragile (*see* Box 4.3),[26] with the potential consequence of the relationship becoming too informal or intimate. One important question for a health professional to ask is 'Whose needs are being met – mine or the patient's?'[27] Particularly vulnerable times for professionals are when they are undergoing relationship or financial problems, have suffered bereavement or are mentally ill. Boundary violations including sexual misconduct are of course reasons to report a health professional to the relevant registration authority in order for them to assess the professional's fitness to practise. However, a patient may disclose sensitive information about a colleague in confidence and not wish the matter to be taken further. The GMC guidelines are clear that doctors have a duty to report professional misconduct,[4] although it may be difficult to proceed with the case without a formal complaint from the patient.

Health professionals often have teaching duties, and therefore have responsibilities arising from these. Boundary violations may occur between health professional and student, and these may be sexual. Of course health professionals often marry other health professionals. The nature of the relationship in the early stages needs to be explored and checked for signs of exploitation. If such a relationship is kept secret, the individuals concerned need to ask themselves why this is important. If there is a guilt-free relationship there should be no concerns about making it public (bar the risk of joking at the expense of either party). Boundary violations may also be fiduciary (i.e. the teacher gives favours to the student for financial gain). For example, teachers may award higher grades or write glowing references that do not entirely reflect the student's actual performance.

RECEIVING GIFTS

Many patients give their doctors and other professional caregivers presents at Christmas or to celebrate other events. These individuals are also likely to give a 'Christmas box' (i.e. present) to their postman/woman and refuse collector. On leaving hospital, many patients donate chocolates and other gifts to the nursing and ward staff. So how should a health professional decide on the propriety of accepting presents from patients?

We need to consider the cost, the nature of the gift, the manner of the giving, and whether the patient expects any benefit or favourable treatment from the giving. A gift may be an attempt to equalize the power differential in the relationship or to seduce the professional, or it may represent a conscious or unconscious bribe.[28] Certainly patients should not be encouraged, or indeed coerced, to give gifts. The GMC advises that doctors 'must not encourage your patients to give, lend or bequeath money or gifts which will directly or indirectly benefit you. You must not put pressure on patients or their families to make donations to other people or organisations.'[4] However, it does not give guidelines about what to do about gifts that are offered spontaneously without solicitation. Refusal of a gift may offend a patient, thus jeopardising the relationship. However, the patient should be aware, as most people who give small presents surely are, that the gift will not affect the manner in which they are treated in the future. When wealthy patients donate large sums of money to institutions as an expression of gratitude for services received, the authorities should make it clear that they will not be treated differently from other patients in the future.

We would doubt whether many health professionals struggle with the dilemma of whether to accept small tokens of appreciation, although they might seek advice from colleagues if a grateful patient exceeded some arbitrary limit of expense (e.g. a bottle of wine might be fine, but a new car would be excessive). However, professional behaviour should mean reflecting on the gift, its cost, its meaning and the implications of accepting or rejecting it. Its meaning could be one of the following:

➤ an expensive gift being a sign that a patient is becoming manic[29]
➤ a farewell gesture from someone who is contemplating suicide
➤ a personal item from a patient who is 'in love' with the doctor.

THE DRUG INDUSTRY

On the subject of gifts we must also consider the relationship between the pharmaceutical companies and doctors. This issue is more pertinent to doctors, as they enjoy much greater freedom to prescribe than other health professionals. It is also relevant to doctor–patient relationships, as patients are unlikely to continue to trust their doctors if they feel that prescribers are influenced by drug company gifts and not by clinical evidence. Medical students and junior doctors are exposed to 'drug lunches' from early in their careers. However much they and more senior doctors deny being influenced by free food and other incentives, we know that the pharmaceutical business would not spend so much money if it did not gain financial rewards.[30] Doctors who accept hospitality from drug companies are more likely to prescribe new drugs and are less likely to prescribe generically and rationally.[31] Estimates suggest that 80–95% of doctors see drug company representatives, despite the evidence that pharmaceutical industry information tends to be overly positive and reduces appropriate prescribing.[32] In fact the number of gifts that a doctor receives correlates with beliefs that drug company representatives have no impact on their prescribing.[31]

Many countries have codes of conduct that stipulate what is a reasonable gift from a drug company. These codes do vary and are often voluntary.[33] In the UK, the Association of the British Pharmaceutical Industry (ABPI) adheres to a voluntary code that is independently regulated by the Prescription Medicine Code of Practice Authority. Gifts to doctors should not exceed £6 in cost and should be relevant to their work, so pens and diaries are allowed, but not music CDs or other home comforts.[34]

However, the entanglement of pharmaceutical companies and doctors extends beyond the giving and receiving of gifts. In January 2008 the Royal College of Physicians in London convened a working party to explore the relationship between doctors and the drug industry, and 'to examine in some detail the political, economic, commercial, organisational, professional and public barriers to creating an ideal relationship.' The ultimate aim was to improve patient care.[35] A major issue is the fact that clinical trials of new drugs are mainly funded by drug companies, leading to bias in reporting and (probably) higher costs.[36]

EMPATHY AND THE PROFESSIONAL–PATIENT RELATIONSHIP

As mentioned above, an empathic consulting style may be more likely to precipitate boundary crossings. However, empathy is also a key attribute and skill in the professional–patient relationship if used properly (and professionally). One definition of empathy is the identification with and understanding of another's situation, feelings and motives. An educationalist's definition is 'The ability to understand your own thoughts and feelings and, by analogy, apply your self-understanding to the service of others, mindful that their thinking and feeling might not match your own.'[37]

Howard Spiro of the Program for Humanities in Medicine at Yale University writes that 'Empathy is the feeling that "I might be you" or "I am you", but is more than just an intellectual identification; empathy must be accompanied by feeling. Sympathy brings compassion, "I want to help you", but empathy brings emotion. Without feeling there is no empathy.'[38]

In relation to professionalism, do we expect our doctors to be objective professionals who do not allow emotion to cloud their judgement? Criticism has been levelled at the empathic doctor on the grounds that such a doctor cannot act objectively and make the best decision: 'Encouraging physicians to cultivate empathy in their relations with patients will undermine their ability to function as wise, understanding doctors who give of themselves in guiding patients through life's concerns and illnesses.'[39] Does good clinical decision making depend on the doctor being distant and unemotional? In the past, doctors would be advised against showing their feelings, particularly in relation to death and dying. A doctor who sheds tears may be viewed as one who cannot continue to practise at an optimal level in the circumstances.

However, it is likely that in order to be therapeutic, doctors must connect with their patients on at least some emotional level in order to motivate them towards healing.[40] But health professionals should be wary of confusing what they would feel in certain situations with what a patient is actually feeling. This tendency has been called 'pseudo-empathy.'[41]

For many people empathy is a natural attribute that may be heightened by personal experience of illness or traumatic events, although even if a health professional has had a similar experience to that of a patient, it will only be similar – it will not be the same. Empathy can also be learned as a technical skill in order to build rapport.[42] There are two stages in the development of empathy:

➤ the understanding and sensitive appreciation of another person's predicament or feelings
➤ the communication of that understanding back to the patient in a supportive manner.[43]

In many professional–patient interactions there may be an understandable lack of empathy. Health professionals may dislike certain patients because of their habits, their past histories or their current behaviour. It is much harder to treat the perpetrator of a violent crime than it is to treat the victim. In such cases patients would expect the doctor or nurse to act 'professionally' – to put their feelings aside and to treat the patient without prejudice. The professional attribute of altruism does not allow for judgements to be made with regard to a patient's treatment on the basis of the aetiology, but only with regard to the patient's likelihood of survival (as in triage).

However, health professionals are human, and their own feelings and experiences will limit their ability to be empathic in certain circumstances. John Salinsky and Paul Sackin, British GPs and course organisers working within a Balint framework of case discussion, have identified defensive over-reactions in consultations that limit empathic responses. They suggest that certain warning signs should alert doctors who are putting up defences against emotional involvement (*see* Box 4.4).[44]

Recognition of such behaviour is important if patient care is not to be compromised. If health professionals feel that they cannot help a patient to the best of their professional ability, they should be honest and admit this. The patient could be referred to a colleague. However, it would be good practice to discuss such feelings with a colleague and to learn from the experience.

BOX 4.4 DEFENSIVE STRATEGIES[44]

- Anxiety
- Feeling irritable
- Being worried about time
- Being withdrawn and aloof
- Being cold and contemptuous
- Anger
- Being careful not to offend
- Overuse of the biomedical model
- Apostolic behaviour
- Talking about health education
- Adhering closely to practice policies
- Feeling too closely identified with the patient

SUMMARY

For most health professionals their relationships with patients are exemplary and therapeutic. However, the potential for transgressing professional behaviour is high, given the power differential, empathic bond and intimate conduct that exist within these relationships. Violence against health professionals is also increasing. Training in these difficult areas is important in order to avoid boundary violations and risk of personal injury.

REFERENCES

1 Brody H. *The Healer's Power.* New Haven, CT: Yale University Press; 1992.
2 Edelstein L. *The Hippocratic Oath: text, translation, and interpretation.* Baltimore, MD: Johns Hopkins University Press; 1943.
3 Leggett A. Origins and development of the injunction prohibiting sexual relationships with patients. *Aust N Z J Psychiatry.* 1995; 29: 586–90.
4 General Medical Council. *Duties of a Doctor: good medical practice.* London: General Medical Council; 1995.
5 General Medical Council. *Maintaining Boundaries.* London: General Medical Council; 2006.
6 General Medical Council. *Professional Conduct and Discipline: fitness to practise.* London: General Medical Council; 1983.
7 Kerridge I, Lowe M, McPhee J. *Ethics and Law for the Health Professions.* 2nd ed. Sydney: The Federation Press; 2005.
8 Searight HR, Campbell DC. Physician–patient sexual contact: ethical and legal issues and clinical guidelines. *J Fam Pract.* 1993; 36: 647–53.
9 Herman J, Gartrell N, Olarte S *et al.* Psychiatrist–patient sexual contact: results of a national survey. II. Psychiatrists' attitudes. *Am J Psychiatry.* 1987; 144: 164–9.

10 Hall KH. Sexualization of the doctor–patient relationship: is it ever ethically permissible? *Fam Pract.* 2001; **18:** 511–15.

11 www.mcnz.org.nz/news/epulse/2006/v8_03.htm (accessed May 2008).

12 www.cgsupport.nhs.uk/downloads/Primary_Care/Chaperone_Framework.pdf (accessed May 2008).

13 Royal College of Obstetricians and Gynaecologists. *Intimate Examinations: report of a working party.* London: RCOG Press; 1997.

14 Rosenthal J, Rymer J, Jones R *et al.* Chaperones for intimate examinations: cross-sectional survey of attitudes and practices of general practitioners. *BMJ.* 2005; **330:** 234–5.

15 Bignell CJ. Chaperones for genital examination. *BMJ.* 1999; **319:** 137–8.

16 Webb R, Opdahl M. Breast and pelvic examinations: easing women's discomfort. *Can Fam Physician.* 1996; **42:** 54–8.

17 BMA Health Policy and Economic Research Unit. *Violence at Work: the experience of UK doctors.* London: British Medical Association; 2003.

18 Cembrowicz S, Rutter S, Wright S. Attacks on doctors and nurses. In: Shepherd J, editor. *Violence in Healthcare.* 2nd ed. Oxford: Oxford University Press; 2001.

19 Levenstein JH, McCracken EC, McWhinney IR *et al.* The patient-centred clinical method. 1. A model for the doctor–patient interaction in family medicine. *Fam Pract.* 1986; **3:** 24–30.

20 Department of Health. *The Patient's Charter.* London: HMSO; 1991.

21 Freidson E. *Professional Dominance.* New York: Atherton; 1970. p. 143.

22 Freidson E. *Profession of Medicine: a study of the sociology of applied knowledge.* New York: Dodd Mead; 1970. pp. 369–70.

23 Lukes S. *Power: a radical view.* London: Macmillan; 1974.

24 Gabbard GO, Nadelson C. Professional boundaries in the physician–patient relationship. *JAMA.* 1995; **273:** 1445–9.

25 Galletly CA. Crossing professional boundaries in medicine: the slippery slope to patient sexual exploitation. *Med J Aust.* 2004; **181:** 380–83.

26 Ellard J. Professional boundaries: the forbidden territories. *Mod Med Aust.* 1998; **July:** 46–9.

27 Corey G, Corey MS, Callanan P. *Issues and Ethics in the Helping Professions.* Pacific Grove, CA: Brooks/Cole; 1998.

28 Lyckhom LJ. Should physicians accept gifts from patients? *JAMA.* 1998; **280:** 1944–6.

29 Spence SA. Patients bearing gifts: are there strings attached? *BMJ.* 2005; **331:** 1527–9.

30 Blumenthal D. Doctors and drug companies. *NEJM.* 2004; **351:** 1185–90.

31 Wazana A. Physicians and the pharmaceutical industry: is a gift ever just a gift? *JAMA.* 2000; **283:** 2655–8.

32 Moynihan R. Who pays for the pizza? Redefining the relationship between doctors and drug companies. I. Entanglement. *BMJ.* 2003; **326:** 1189–92.

33 Wager E. How to dance with porcupines: roles and guidelines on doctors' relationships with drug companies. *BMJ.* 2003; **326:** 1196–8.

34 www.abpi.org.uk (accessed May 2008).

35 Ferriman A. Royal College sets up working party to improve relations between doctors and drug industry; www.bmj.com/cgi/content/full/336/7634/14-a (accessed February 2008).

36 Godlee F. Doctors and the drug industry; www.bmj.com/cgi/content/full/336/7634/0 (accessed February 2008).

37 Arnold R. *Empathic Intelligence: teaching, learning, relating.* Sydney: UNSW Press; 2005.

38 Spiro HM. Empathy: an introduction. In: Spiro H, Curnen MGM, Peschel E *et al.*, editors. *Empathy and the Practice of Medicine.* New Haven, CT: Yale University Press; 1993. pp. 1–6.

39 Landau RL. . . . And the least of these is empathy. In: Spiro H, Curnen MGM, Peschel E *et al.*, editors. *Empathy and the Practice of Medicine.* New Haven, CT: Yale University Press; 1993. pp. 103–9.

40 Coulehan JL. Tenderness and steadiness: emotions in medical practice. *Lit Med.* 1995; **14:** 222–36.

41 Rosenfield PJ, Jones L. Striking a balance: training medical students to provide empathic care. *Med Educ.* 2004; **38:** 927–33.

42 Platt VW, Keller VF. Empathic communication: a teachable and learnable skill. *J Gen Intern Med.* 1994; **9:** 222–6.

43 Silverman J, Kurtz S, Draper J. *Skills for Communicating with Patients.* Oxford: Radcliffe Medical Press; 1998. pp. 83–4.

44 Salinsky J, Sackin P. *What Are You Feeling Doctor? Identifying and avoiding defensive patterns in the consultation.* Oxford: Radcliffe Medical Press; 2000.

CHAPTER 5

Communication and its relationship with professionalism

This chapter explores:
- the different contexts in which professional communication is important
- failures of communication and their relationship to litigation
- barriers to good communication
- communication and consent
- teamwork
- interprofessional communication and education
- issues relating to confidentiality.

> . . . a map of the communications within a particular profession . . . will soon reveal how limited is the extent of what is taught in formal education. There is even a suspicion that some communication capabilities are worsened rather than improved by the process of professionalisation.
>
> *Michael Eraut, 1994*[1]

Good communication is fundamental to all areas of professionalism. Furthermore, the ever increasing number of books on this subject is testimony to the importance of communication in twenty-first-century life. As well as the obvious issue of one-to-one (patient–doctor) communication, there are skills to be learned relating to written, group, team and interprofessional interactions. In addition, in this electronic age, we need to think about the advantages and perils of email and the Internet, and newer small mobile technologies such as personal digital assistants and smart phones, which are developing rapidly and which have huge potential in healthcare. Moreover, we need to recognise the power of the media, particularly television, in influencing doctor, health professional and patient behaviour. There is also a necessity to understand and be understood by people for whom English is not their first language, or who have other difficulties relating to ease of communication, such as physical impairment, learning difficulty or mental health problems. New communication challenges face both doctors and patients, including increasing expectations of a more active patient role in care, the burgeoning of information on the Internet (World Wide Web) and the evolution of new web technologies (e.g. social networking), communicating about risk and benefit, the fact that research findings often reach the public via the Internet or other media before the profession hear about them, and so on.

THE ART OF COMMUNICATION

A hallmark of professional behaviour and skill is the ability to communicate with a diverse group of people and to make oneself understood. For this reason, professional training now devotes more curricular time to 'communication skills' training, including its assessment. Indeed a core curriculum for communication in medical education has been published.[2] Often in medical school such training focuses on communication between professional and patient, but more recently the focus has begun to broaden – for example, to address communication with peers and other professionals. However, there are many situations and diverse interactions that require good communication, each of which has its own potential pitfalls (*see* Box 5.1). Not all of these are covered in training at present.

BOX 5.1 PROFESSIONAL COMMUNICATION

HP (health professional)–patient communication
● Consultation: face-to-face in a wide variety of contexts
● Consultation: telephone
● Written
● Email
● Appropriate use of computer in the consultation

HP–patient's family/carers
● Face-to-face (including 'third party' where patient is not present)
● Written
● Electronic

HP–HP (same profession) (e.g. doctor–doctor)
- Professional (e.g. referral)
- Case discussion
- Handover
- Seeking or giving advice
- Interactions with junior or senior colleagues
- Appraisal and mentoring
- Treating a doctor as a patient
- Verbal
- Telephone
- Written

HP–HP (different profession) (e.g. doctor–physiotherapist)
- Referral
- Seeking or giving advice
- Handover
- Case discussion

Writing medical records (paper or electronic)

Legal
- Reports
- Court appearances

Communication with the media

Communication with the police

Dealing with complaints
- Against oneself, including admitting error and apologising
- Against others

Whistleblowing

Conflict resolution and negotiation skills

Running/chairing meetings
- Facilitating a small group educational meeting
- Practice meetings
- Committees
- Video or tele-conferencing

Presentations to a large group of professionals
- Lectures
- Case presentations

Teaching
- One-to-one
- Group
- Bedside or clinic
- Giving feedback
- Lay people

Writing for publication
- Papers/articles
- Reports
- Letters

IS THERE A PROBLEM?

A few years ago the Lothian University Hospital Trusts in Scotland carried out a survey of patients to find out their views on communication. Almost two-thirds complained about a lack of involvement in decisions about their care, and the fact that they were given no information about resuming normal activities after discharge. One-third of respondents said that they had been given no explanation of test results, nor had they had the opportunity to talk to a doctor. With regard to teamwork, 23% of respondents complained that doctors and nurses said different things.[3] As NHS Scotland states, there is no reason to suppose that the results would be different elsewhere in the country (and presumably not in the rest of the UK either).

The 2002 Commonwealth Health Fund International Health Policy Survey of Sicker Adults found that around 50% of patients in the five countries surveyed felt that their regular doctor did not ask for their ideas and opinions about treatment and care (the figures ranged from 47% in the USA and New Zealand to 67% in the UK).[4] Finally, a 2005 report from Picker Institute Europe, based on the results of 15 national patient surveys conducted in the UK between 1998 and 2004, highlighted a number of problem areas. For example, 21% of outpatients and 26% of Accident and Emergency patients said that staff did not always listen carefully to what they were saying, 28% of inpatients said that doctors talked in front of them, and 35% of mental health patients and 32% of outpatients said that they did not receive clear explanations about the risks and side-effects of medication. There had apparently been little improvement in any of these areas since previous surveys.[5] A more recent Picker Institute report, published in 2007, showed little change in the number of NHS patients who were happy with the listening skills and explanations of their doctors, but both patients and their carers complained about the lack of information they receive about how to look after themselves – information that they want.[6] Moreover, 32% of patients in primary care and 48% of those in hospital said that they had not been sufficiently involved in treatment decisions.[6] Clearly there is a problem.

Research into the effects of good and bad communication is plentiful.[7] In summary, good communication leads to more accurate diagnosis, greater patient satisfaction, a greater likelihood that the patient will adhere to treatment decisions, a reduction in stress and anxiety, better quality of life and an improvement in the doctor's own well-being.

MISCOMMUNICATION

Professional knowledge brings with it a jargon all of its own. The specialised body of knowledge that belongs to a profession has its own inherent vocabulary. Students and apprentices entering at the lowest levels of the professional hierarchy soon pick up this profession-specific language. Jargon – the original meaning of which was 'gibberish' – is not necessarily a quicker way of communicating (think of the eight syllables of myocardial infarction compared with the three of heart attack), but may convey an aura of mystique and learning to the non-initiated. Although many professionals simply forget that not all patients are conversant in medical matters, such jargon may also be used as a security blanket, particularly by junior and/or insecure doctors. It may even be used deliberately to confuse the non-professional, being seen as an important distinguishing feature of the trained professional: 'Isn't he clever, talking with all those long words?' Eliot Freidson, an American sociologist and notable critic of the medical profession, suggested in 1970 that doctors deliberately withhold information from patients in order to maintain their professional dominance and power.[8] Giving information in unintelligible terms to the layperson could be construed as the same process. Freidson argued that such behaviour stemmed from doctors' 'splendid isolation' from society at large, and led to the exertion of an unreasonable level of social control.[9] In the previous era of paternalism and 'doctor knows best', not only were difficult words perhaps used to keep patients ill informed, but names of drugs and ailments were also hidden – for example, the bottle of medicine that was simply labelled 'The mixture', and the diagnosis of 'erythema ab igne' for the redness of skin caused by sitting too close to the fire. Although Freidson was writing nearly 40 years ago, his observations still ring true.

Latin, as in the latter example, is still in use today, while shorthand and illegible writing all help to form a barrier between doctor and patient. The poor handwriting of doctors is legendary, although computerised records and prescriptions have helped to overcome this method of obfuscation. Shorthand and the ubiquitous TLA (three-letter acronym) are dangerous, as they confuse health professionals as well. For example, PID may be both prolapsed intervertebral disc and pelvic inflammatory disease, and IUD may be intrauterine device or intrauterine death. Acronyms have also been used pejoratively to describe or categorise patients – for example, NFN (Normal for Norfolk), etc.

Acronyms and abbreviations abound in health service management. Search the Internet and you will find a plethora of websites designed as jargon busters. The NHS seems to run several of these. Box 5.2 lists some of the abbreviations and their decipherment on one such site.[10] The problem is that even with the words written out in full, it is not always obvious what is being written about. Moreover, even everyday words may confuse patients if they are used in an unusual context or without adequate explanation[11] – for example, 'threatened abortion', 'bad fats' and 'benign growth.'

BOX 5.2 SOME PROFESSIONAL JARGON AND ABBREVIATIONS

ABPI	Association of the British Pharmaceutical Industry
AHPs	Allied health professionals
CDO	Chief Dental Officer
CMO	Chief Medical Officer
CNO	Chief Nursing Officer
CHAI	Commission of Healthcare Audit and Inspection
CHC	Community Health Council
CHPO	Chief Health Professions Officer
CPPIH	Commission for Patient and Public Involvement in Health
CREST	Clinical Resource Efficiency Support Team
HAZ	Health Action Zone
HIMP	Health Improvement Programme
MHRA	Medicines and Healthcare Products Regulatory Agency
PCO	Primary Care Organisation
SHA	Strategic Health Authority
tPCT	Teaching Primary Care Trust

For many patients the letters after a health professional's name are meaningless. It is not necessarily the case that the more there are, the 'better' the professional is. There is endless confusion about 'Dr' and 'Mr' for medical professionals, and even more so if a nurse is a doctor due to having a PhD. On the wards a variety of health professionals interact with patients. Although all are required to wear name badges, the different uniforms and changing shifts confuse patients who are already vulnerable due to illness.

BARRIERS TO GOOD COMMUNICATION

The British Medical Association has identified both personal and organisational factors that are barriers to communication (*see* Box 5.3).[12]

BOX 5.3 BARRIERS TO GOOD COMMUNICATION[11]

Personal barriers
- Lack of skill and training
- Poor language skills (English as a second language)
- Lack of understanding that clear communication is important
- Negative attitudes to communication
- Providing explanations for patients being seen as a low priority
- Lack of time
- Tiredness
- Stress

Organisational barriers
- Pressure of work
- Emphasis on throughput of patients
- Culture of not involving patients in decisions

Some of these barriers may be overcome by training programmes, particularly experiential learning sessions with the use of role play and videotaping, working with simulated patients and feedback. Assessment of communication skills shows that an institution or organisation is committed to good communication at all levels of the health service.

Communication with people whose first language is not English can be a difficult challenge, both for the health professional and for the patient. Health professional and patient need to consider whether a therapeutic interaction is feasible, depending on the extent of any language barrier. This may be difficult to assess, as a patient may appear to be fairly fluent in English but lack understanding of colloquialisms, technical terms or jargon that the doctor uses. Checking understanding is therefore crucial.

Both health professional and patient may become frustrated due to lack of understanding, thus reinforcing prejudice and leading to poor care. The patient may already feel isolated and culture shocked, and illness adds to their feelings of helplessness. Health professionals should avoid pretending to understand when they do not. Patients may also nod and express understanding even if they are confused. In some cultures people will not interrupt or question a person in a position of power, and they view a doctor or nurse in this way. It is important to summarise advice and to give appropriate written information in the person's own language. Ideally an interpreter should be present, preferably someone who is not a family member, although in reality this is a common scenario. Interpreters should work in such a way that both the effect and the meaning of words and phrases are conveyed. If possible they should have relevant cultural knowledge and an appropriate professional background.[13] Even if a suitable interpreter is available, there may be still be a lack of understanding. Interpreters may subtly alter meaning, particularly when a patient's ideas and concerns, or less concrete concepts, are being discussed. Problems may arise, for example, with regard to confidentiality when the interpreter is from the same community as the patient (which is almost always the case in small communities). Finally, although codes of practice for interpreters exist, they may not be adhered to on every occasion.

Communication is obviously not just about one's 'mother tongue', but is also influenced by more subtle cultural differences, including kinship, social support, health beliefs and explanatory models of illness, religious ideology and healthcare expectations. Moreover, health professionals must learn that patients' identities are not limited by a definition of their race, ethnicity or culture. These identities change over time, and are often in a state of flux due to the impact of new social movements, globalisation and racism.[14] Finally, it is important to be alert to stereotyping, since there may be as much difference and diversity *within* a particular group as there is between groups.

OUTCOMES OF POOR COMMUNICATION

The professional literature includes many research papers relating to communication – the results of poor communication, how to improve interpersonal skills, and how patient satisfaction and other outcomes are linked to communication. The problem is that the papers keep on being published because the problems still remain. Despite the increase in training and recognition of the problem, doctors' behaviour (or at least the public's perception of it) does not appear to have changed much. Litigation against doctors is often related to failure of some aspect of communication.

Wendy Levinson and her North American colleagues showed in 1997 that doctors who were sued spent on average 3.5 to 4 minutes less time with patients. Doctors with no claims against them used more humour in consultations, they touched patients more when comforting them (e.g. held the patient's hand), and they sat down and provided better explanations while also checking the patient's understanding of what had been said.[15] In Australia, in 1999, a survey of 500 patients who had complained about their medical care showed that rudeness and poor communication were factors in 22% of the complaints.[16] The majority of medical errors may be traced back to poor communication.[17]

In the UK, the Bristol Inquiry into the performance of paediatric heart surgeons showed that lack of communication was a factor in the poor outcomes, including communication between different professionals caring for the patients.[18] Some of the recommendations relating to communication are listed in Box 5.4.

BOX 5.4 RECOMMENDATIONS FROM THE BRISTOL INQUIRY[18]

- Involve patients/parents in decisions.
- Keep patients/parents informed.
- Improve communication with patients/parents.
- Provide patients and their families with counselling and support.
- Obtain informed consent for all procedures and processes.
- Elicit feedback from patients and listen to their views.
- Be open and candid when adverse events occur.

COMMUNICATING WITH PATIENTS AND THE PUBLIC

Although communication skills training starts with the fundamentals of interpersonal interactions (introductions, body language, information gathering, information sharing, empathy, etc.), more experienced students and health professionals also need to develop a culture of patient partnership that includes involving patients in decisions about their healthcare. Patient partnership has become part of UK national policy as defined by the National Health Service Executive.[19] Angela Coulter, Chief Executive of Picker Institute Europe, is an expert on patient partnership,[20] and advocates moving away from the often still pervasive model of medical paternalism towards a model that encourages patient self-reliance and empowerment. She lists ways in which patients are able to become more involved in their own management (*see* Box 5.5).[21]

BOX 5.5 STRATEGIES TO ENABLE PATIENT INVOLVEMENT IN HEALTHCARE[21]

- Health professionals to recognise patients' expertise, values and preferences.
- Patients being offered informed choice, not passive consent.
- Training in shared decision making (for both health professionals and patients).
- Evidence-based decision aids for patients.
- Public education in interpreting clinical evidence.
- Patient access to electronic health records.
- Surveys of patients' experience in order to prioritise quality improvements.
- Openness and empathy with patients and their families after medical errors have occurred.
- Public access to comparative data on quality and outcomes.

Many of these strategies for patient involvement relate to communication in one form or another. Sharing and discussing information about investigation and treatment (including risks and benefits), negotiation about management, frank disclosure of why certain treatment options are not available (due to cost or waiting lists), and exploration with patients and families about critical incidents, adverse outcomes and medical errors – including apologising – are all interactions that require skill just as much as more traditional areas such as 'breaking bad news'.

Step 5 of the (UK) National Patient Safety Agency (NPSA) *Seven Steps to Patient Safety* is 'Involve and communicate with patients and the public.'[22] In particular, the NPSA recommends apologising to patients and carers following any adverse events – a shift away from the previous approach to management of critical incidents. 'Central to the NPSA's strategy to improve patient safety is our commitment to improving communication between healthcare organisations and patient and/or carers when a patient is moderately harmed, severely harmed or has died as a result of a patient safety incident . . . this communication is known as being open.'[23]

The paternalistic doctor, wishing to protect his patient from uncertainty and the possibility of failure of treatment, may be unhappy about the move towards patient partnership with its tinge of consumerism. The consummate professional, faced with a demanding patient who is requesting information about every conceivable side-effect of a drug, may act the part of information provider while believing that such openness is really not in the patient's best interests. The question is whether it matters what the doctor or health professional really thinks, so long as they act in the spirit of patient partnership. Should we be measured by what we do (behaviour) rather than by what we believe (attitude)?

BEHAVIOUR AND ATTITUDES

A 'rough and ready' description of attitudes is 'a mixture of beliefs, thoughts and feelings that predispose a person to respond, in a positive or negative way, to objects, people, processes or institutions.'[24] In the UK, the General Medical Council has defined one of the goals of undergraduate medical education as follows: 'the student should acquire and demonstrate attitudes necessary for the achievement of high standards of medical practice . . . in relation to the provision of care of individuals.'[25] Appropriate attitudes underpinning practice are further reinforced in *Good Medical Practice*,[26] and are fundamental to most modern definitions or conceptualisations of 'professionalism' (*see* Chapter 1). Attitudes may be inferred from behaviour, but in practice the correlation between observed behaviour and attitudes is not always high.[27]

This implies that health professionals do act a role within some patient interactions. We have to be honest – there are some patients with whom we find it difficult to empathise, or who make us angry or defensive. Health professionals cannot like every patient, agree with the decisions that patients make, or remain unaffected by what are seen as unreasonable demands. The way that practitioners relate to patients is also influenced by their own experiences and 'baggage' (both professional and personal), and by their state of physical and mental health at the time of the interaction. Feeling tired or ill, or working following an argument at home or while under investigation for a complaint, affects responses to patients and thus communication with them. The best actors may be able to interact at the highest level of professional competence under such circumstances, but many will find it difficult to engage fully with the patients' needs. In the same way, such stresses may cause the usual professional façade to slip and one's true attitudes to be revealed. For example, a tired nurse may show their irritability towards a patient who refuses to accept any of the professional advice on offer, or a racist doctor who normally treats patients equally may, under pressure, make a derogatory comment either to the patient or to a colleague.

Thus, although professional behaviour is important, as it is what patients and peers observe, we should also strive to measure professional attitudes, as 'negative' attitudes may not always be kept concealed. The assessment of attitudes is a relatively new area in medical education, but is recognised as an important dimension of professionalism and a key aspect of ensuring competence for the future doctor.[28] Methods that may be used to assess attitudes include interviews,[24] direct observation,[29] written tests and portfolios,[30] and self-report methods such as questionnaires.[24] An interesting aspect of the assessment of attitudes is that those of medical students do change during their education, although often in the direction of a decrease in humanistic values and empathy.[31] Perhaps this is a reason for assessing attitudes regularly during a health professional's career.

INFORMED CHOICE AND INFORMED CONSENT

Modern medical practice recognises the necessity for patients to be given the full range of evidence about any management they are considering undertaking. In contrast to paternalism, the 'informed model'[32] of professional–patient interaction involves the health professional adopting a completely neutral stance. The patient is given a range of options about which the professional expresses no opinions. This model may be seen as a move towards increased patient autonomy. The rationale is that the patient should be free to decide on a management plan without being influenced by the health professional's preferences or bias.[33] Communication within this framework is still largely one-sided. Instead of the professional having overall control over the decision, the onus is put on the patient without any practical or emotional support.

BOX 5.6 CHARACTERISTICS OF SHARED DECISION MAKING[35]

- Both the patient and the doctor are involved.
- Both parties share information.
- Both parties take steps to build a consensus about the preferred treatment.
- Doctor and patient reach an agreement on the treatment to implement.

To some this goes too far: 'Too often autonomous patients and families are asked to make critical medical decisions on the basis of neutrally presented statistics, as free as possible from the contaminating influences of physicians.'[34] Shared decision making is preferred as the middle ground. Charles and colleagues have defined a model of shared decision making that has four main characteristics (*see* Box 5.6).[35] The commitment of both health professional and patient to engage in the process is crucial, and requires a high degree of skill in communication.

Truly informed consent, whether to an invasive investigation or operation, to intimate examinations, or to involvement in teaching or research, is a further step along the path of professional–patient interaction. It involves both verbal and written communication. Individual doctors are responsible for informing patients about the risks of procedures, whereas the consent form itself is often the product of a committee who have received legal advice on what generic information to include on the form.

In British law, consent to treatment is required because without it the health professional may be open to a charge of battery (i.e. trespass) of the patient. The consequence of this is that doctors only have to give a broad description of the impending procedure, which the patient has to understand.[36] However, whether *informed* consent has been obtained, in the sense that patients have been informed of risks, may also be used in cases of medical negligence. In the USA, informed consent is based on the 'reasonable person standard (prudent patient test).' This concept, which was established in 1972, states that a doctor's decision about whether a patient should have been informed of a risk is based on whether a reasonable person in that patient's position would want to be informed.[37] In the UK there is the 'prudent doctor test', which states that a doctor is not negligent if he or she acts in accordance with a responsible body of medical opinion.[36] However, whichever test is applied, a patient's signature on a form does not provide evidence that they received an adequate explanation of the procedure and its risks. The doctor has a duty to ensure that the patient understands. Failure of communication in this respect leaves the doctor open to litigation if there is a subsequent problem. A valid consent has three elements (*see* Box 5.7).[36]

BOX 5.7 VALID INFORMED CONSENT[36]

- The patient must have sufficient understanding, variously described as mental capacity or competence, to make the decision.
- The patient must consent to (or refuse) the treatment of his or her own free will, with no duress or undue influence.
- The patient must have been given sufficient information about the proposed treatment.

INTERPROFESSIONAL COMMUNICATION AND COMMUNICATION WITHIN TEAMS

The modern healthcare service is about teamwork – health professionals working together to achieve better outcomes for patients, using their professional expertise to complement each other's roles. Often there may be not only several doctors looking after one patient, but also nurses, physiotherapists, occupational therapists, etc. Pharmacists, receptionists and complementary therapists also have roles in certain circumstances. In these days of super-specialisation and increasingly complex healthcare interventions, one health professional is unlikely to have all the knowledge and skills necessary to look after every patient.

One of the hallmarks of good teamwork is communication. Often the various health professionals involved in a patient's care do not meet face-to-face on a regular basis. Therefore methods of keeping in touch other than personal meetings are important. Systems need to be in place to cope with the complexity and heavy workload of all concerned, which often means that various team members are rarely in the same place at the same time. For this reason, leadership and accountability are important. Tasks in patient care should not be repeated by different professionals. Moreover, all of those involved in management should not give conflicting advice to patients. Communication channels therefore need to be open and functioning.

A study of communication behaviours in a hospital setting in the UK found several examples of inefficiencies with regard to team communication: 'For example, a senior consultant tried to transfer a patient to another's team by delegating the request, involving at least two intermediaries. By the time the second consultant received the message, it was substantially distorted and had the potential to endanger the patient.'[38] We are all familiar with the situation of waiting on the end of the phone while trying to contact a health professional for advice or referral. We leave a message. The health professional rings back when we are seeing a patient. Do we have the conversation there and then, ask the professional to ring back later, or ask the patient to leave? All of these options are unsatisfactory solutions. This study concluded that individual health professionals need to consider carefully the effects of their communication behaviour, particularly what the researchers called 'interruptive behaviours', on their own efficiency and effectiveness as well as on that of others.[38]

No longer is the doctor automatically the team leader, although this is still commonly the case. As with the doctor–patient relationship itself and the demise of paternalism in favour of partnership, professional teams should work as partners. There must be respect for different views and negotiation, often involving the patient, with regard to the best management plan for the optimum outcome. Each member of the team has a duty of care to the patient and to the other members of the team. Professional teamwork is about mutual respect and making the best use of each member's expertise and insights.

Respectful behaviour is demonstrated by listening to other members and valuing their input. If members disagree, which is bound to happen frequently, they should try to resolve their differences through dialogue and with evidence, rather than going it alone or undermining each other with other staff.

THE DYSFUNCTIONAL TEAM

Three conditions define a functioning team:
➤ clear objectives that are known to all members
➤ members work closely together to achieve these objectives
➤ regular meetings to review team effectiveness and discuss how it can be improved.

Health professionals who identify themselves as working in teams but who do not meet all of these criteria have been defined as working within 'pseudo-teams', and they report lower safety at work and less job satisfaction.[39]

A poor team may work badly for a number of reasons. There may be no designated leader or co-ordinator of tasks. There may be personal disagreements between members. Although such personal feelings should not affect professional duties, they often lead to poor performance and stress, thereby affecting patient care and the morale of the whole team.

If the more senior members of the team are not open to suggestion and feedback, junior members will find it difficult to interact with them. Juniors may be unable to challenge the views or actions of their superiors even if they attempt to do so in a respectful way. On the other hand, some senior staff find it difficult to criticise their trainees or other team members constructively, and either resort to bullying or let poor performance go unchecked. As health professionals ascend the promotion ladder on the basis of clinical expertise, assessments and/or research results, they are not always trained in personnel management. They may be wonderful communicators with patients but be unable to delegate, or to trust other professionals, or to mentor juniors in a supportive and educational manner.

Once a team becomes dysfunctional, patient care is likely to suffer, and this is obviously not to be tolerated. If the team leader is able to sit down with the team members either as a group or individually and diagnose and rectify the problem, the team may be able to function effectively again. If this is not possible, or the team has lost faith in the leader, an outside consultant should be invited to help the team to diagnose and evaluate its problems.

INTERPROFESSIONAL EDUCATION

As professionals do not always collaborate well together in clinical practice, interprofessional education (IPE) has been suggested as a means of rectifying this situation. IPE involves the health professions learning with, from and about each other.[40] There are many IPE initiatives in place both nationally and internationally. A major problem at present is whether these projects – at undergraduate and postgraduate levels, and in the workplace – are achieving any change in the way in which professionals do work and communicate together. A Cochrane Review published in 2000 concluded that 'despite finding a large body of literature on the evaluation of IPE, these studies lacked the methodological rigour needed to begin to convincingly understand the impact of IPE on professional practice and/or healthcare outcomes.'[41] More recently, the Best Evidence Medical Education (BEME) Group has published a systematic review which concludes that 'IPE is generally well received, enabling knowledge and skills necessary for collaborative working to be learnt.'[42]

BOX 5.8 MODEL OF OUTCOMES FOR IPE[43]

1.	Reaction	Learners' views on the learning experience and its interprofessional nature
2a.	Modification of attitudes/ behaviour	Changes in reciprocal attitudes or perceptions between groups
2b.	Acquisition of knowledge/skills	Including knowledge and skills linked to interprofessional collaboration
3.	Behavioural change	Transfer of interprofessional learning to practice setting and changed professional practice
4a.	Change in organisational practice	Wider changes in organisation and delivery of care
4b.	Benefits to patients/ clients	Improvements in health or well-being of patients/clients

---

The UK Centre for the Advancement of Interprofessional Education (CAIPE) has developed a model of outcomes for IPE, derived from Kirkpatrick (*see* Box 5.8).[43,44] Its critical review of IPE evaluations commissioned by the then

Learning and Teaching Support Network (LTSN), now the Higher Education Academy Subject Centre for Medicine, Dentistry and Veterinary Science, looked at IPE in practice and found that most studies reported outcomes at more than one of these levels.[44] However, there is a need for more prospective studies with longer-term follow-up to establish the place and role of IPE in professional curricula.

CONFIDENTIALITY: BE CAREFUL WITH WHOM YOU COMMUNICATE

The GMC has defined one of the duties of a doctor as being to 'respect and protect confidential information.'[45] The *Oxford Dictionary of English* defines the word 'confidential' as 'intended to be kept secret.'[46] In the public eye, confidentiality is one of the hallmarks of the professional. Patients do not expect their private business and embarrassing conditions to be discussed outside the consulting room. Yet personal details of illness are divulged on a regular basis in the media by hospital spokespersons speaking about their famous patients. The final days of Pope John Paul II were hardly secret, and his slow dying was hardly kept confidential. In the past, medical journals carried photographs of patients and case histories in the belief that few laypeople would have access to them. These days, written permission is needed before such material can be published, and names are obviously changed to help to preserve the anonymity of the individuals concerned. So what constitutes confidential information and with whom may we discuss it in these days of teamwork and the information highway?

The GMC's booklet *Confidentiality: Protecting and Providing Information* offers a good overview of the subject. It states on page 1 that 'Doctors hold information about patients which is private and sensitive. This information must not be given to others unless the patient consents or you can justify the disclosure.'[47] It should not be assumed that patients would expect other healthcare team members to have access to their records. In common law, personal information may only be disclosed without the patient's consent if it is in the public interest to do so. Public interest would imply that there would be greater harm to other parties than to the patient if certain information was not divulged. Confidentiality may be broken if patients or others are at serious risk of injury or death.

Why patients should expect professionals to keep secrets in this way is interesting. The assumption is that patients would not be open and honest about their problems if they thought that other people would be privy to such information. Yet in these days of 'reality TV' it seems that certain people are not only happy to talk about their lives, successes and dishonesty, but also that they do not mind the minutiae of their day-to-day existence being broadcast live to a global audience.

The ethical dilemmas relating to confidentiality are numerous. Normally a professional would not talk to a relative about a family member's illness, but if that family member is unable to give consent due to being unconscious or demented, it would seem churlish for the professional not to tell the relatives about the likely course of the illness. Here the health professional needs to remember that he or she might have to justify the disclosure if at a later date the patient complains about it. In fact the law does not sanction the disclosure of information even to blood relatives unless the health professional is able to prove implied or tacit consent.[36]

Therefore communicating about patients to third parties needs careful consideration and attention to detail. Health professionals often release tension by discussing cases and sharing anecdotes. It should be remembered that patients are often easy to identify, or a health professional listening to such details may be a relative or connected to the patient in some way.

SUMMARY

Good communication skills are an important attribute for any health professional. Effective and ethical communication is necessary between professional and patient and also between professional and professional. Both verbal and written communication skills are necessary. Teamwork is not possible without communication between members. However, attention must also be given to confidentiality and to the choice of individuals with whom information is to be shared.

REFERENCES

1 Eraut M. *Developing Professional Knowledge and Competence*. London: Routledge Falmer; 1994.
2 Schofield T. A curriculum for communication in medical education. In: Macdonald E, editor. *Difficult Conversations in Medicine*. Oxford: Oxford University Press; 2004. pp. 209–21.
3 NHS Scotland. *Talking Matters: developing the communication skills of doctors*. Edinburgh: Scottish Executive; 2003.
4 Blendon RJ, Schoen C, Des Roches C *et al.* Common concerns amid diverse systems: health care experiences in five countries. *Health Affairs.* 2003; **22**: 106–21.
5 Coulter A. *Is the NHS Getting Better or Worse?* Oxford: Picker Institute Europe; 2005; www.pickereurope.org (accessed February 2008).
6 Richards N, Coulter A. *Is the NHS Becoming More Patient-Centred?* Oxford: Picker Institute Europe; 2007; www.pickereurope.org (accessed February 2008).

7 Silverman J, Kurtz S, Draper J. *Skills for Communicating with Patients*. 2nd ed. Oxford: Radcliffe Publishing; 2005.

8 Freidson E. *Professional Dominance*. New York: Atherton; 1970.

9 Freidson E. *Profession of Medicine: a study of the sociology of applied knowledge*. New York: Dodd Mead; 1970.

10 www.jbmedical.com/orac-grpn-nhsjargon.htm (accessed October 2005).

11 Hadlow J, Pitts M. The understanding of common terms by doctors, nurses and patients. *Soc Sci Med*. 1991; **32**: 193–6.

12 British Medical Association. *Communication Skills Education for Doctors*. London: British Medical Association; 2002.

13 Robinson L. Intercultural communication in a therapeutic setting. In: Coker N, editor. *Racism in Medicine*. London: King's Fund; 2001. pp. 191–210.

14 Pfeffer N. Theories of race, ethnicity and culture. *BMJ*. 1998; **317**: 1381–4.

15 Levinson W, Roter DL, Mullooly JP *et al*. Physician–patient communication: the relationship with malpractice claims among primary care physicians and surgeons. *JAMA*. 1997; **277**: 553–9.

16 Daniel AE, Burn RJ, Hororik S. Patients' complaints about medical practice. *Med J Aust*. 1999; **170**: 598–602.

17 Haynes K, Thomas M. *Clinical Risk Management in Primary Care*. Oxford: Radcliffe Publishing; 2005.

18 Bristol Royal Infirmary Inquiry. *Learning from Bristol: the report of the public inquiry into children's heart surgery at the Bristol Royal Infirmary, 1984–1995*. London: The Stationery Office, 2001; www.bristol-inquiry.org.uk (accessed April 2008).

19 NHS Executive. *Patient Partnership: building a collaborative strategy*. Leeds: NHS Executive; 1996.

20 Coulter A. Paternalism or partnership? *BMJ*. 1999; **319**: 719–20.

21 Coulter A. After Bristol: putting patients at the centre. *BMJ*. 2002; **324**: 648–51.

22 National Patient Safety Agency. *Seven Steps to Patient Safety: the full reference guide*; www.npsa.nhs.uk/sevensteps (accessed May 2008).

23 National Patient Safety Agency. *Being Open: communicating patient safety incidents with patients and their carers*. London: National Patient Safety Agency; 2005.

24 Brown G, Manogue M, Rohlin M. Assessing attitudes in dental education: is it worthwhile? *Br Dent J*. 2002; **193**: 703–7.

25 General Medical Council. *Tomorrow's Doctors*. London: General Medical Council; 1993.

26 www.gmc-uk.org/guidance/good_medical_practice/index.asp (accessed May 2008).

27 Kaplan RM. Behaviour as the central outcome of health care. *Am Psychol*. 1990; **45**: 1211–20.

28 Shumway JM, Harden RM. AMEE Guide No. 25: The assessment of learning outcomes for the competent and reflective physician. *Med Teach*. 2003; **25**: 569–84.

29 Phelan S, Obenshain SS, Galey WR. Evaluation of the non-cognitive professional traits of medical students. *Acad Med*. 1993; **68**: 799–803.

30 Rethans J-J, Sturmans F, Drop R *et al*. Assessment of the performance of general practitioners by the use of standardized (simulated) patients. *Br J Gen Pract*. 1991; **41**: 97–9.

31 Wolf TM, Balson PM, Faucett JM *et al*. A retrospective study of attitude change during medical education. *Med Educ*. 1989; **23**: 19–23.

32 Tomlinson T. The physician's influence on patients' choices. *Theor Med.* 1986; **7:** 105–21.

33 Brodky H. Autonomy revisited: progress in medical ethics: discussion paper. *J R Soc Med.* 1985; **78:** 380–87.

34 Quill TE, Brody H. Physician recommendations and patient autonomy: finding a balance between physician power and patient choice. *Ann Intern Med.* 1996; **125:** 763–9.

35 Charles C, Gafni A, Whelan T. Shared decision-making in the medical encounter: what does it mean? (or it takes at least two to tango). *Soc Sci Med.* 1997; **44:** 681–92.

36 Stauch M, Wheat K, Tingle J. *Sourcebook on Medical Law.* 2nd ed. London: Cavendish Publishing Limited; 2002.

37 Mazur DJ. Influence of the law on risk and informed consent. *BMJ.* 2003; **327:** 731–4.

38 Coiera E, Tombs V. Communication behaviours in a hospital setting: an observational study. *BMJ.* 1998; **316:** 673–6.

39 Dawson JF, Yan X, West MA. *Positive and Negative Effects of Team Working in Healthcare: real and pseudo-teams and their impact on safety.* Birmingham: Aston University; 2007.

40 Barr H. *Interprofessional Education 1997–2000: a review.* London: UK Centre for Advancement of Interprofessional Education (CAIPE); 2000.

41 Zwarenstein M, Reeves S, Barr H *et al.* Interprofessional education: effects on professional practice and health care outcomes. In: *The Cochrane Database of Systematic Reviews. Issue 3.* Oxford: Update Software; 2000.

42 Hammick M, Freeth, D, Koppel I *et al.* A best evidence systematic review of interprofessional education. *Med Teach.* 2007; **29:** 735–751.

43 Kirkpatrick DI. *Evaluating Training Programs: the four levels.* San Francisco, CA: Berrett-Koehler; 1994.

44 Freeth D, Hammick M, Koppel I *et al. A Critical Review of Evaluations of Interprofessional Education.* London: LTSN for Health Sciences and Practice; 2002.

45 General Medical Council. *The Duties of a Doctor.* London: General Medical Council; 2002.

46 Soanes C, Stevenson A, editors. *Oxford Dictionary of English.* 2nd ed. Oxford: Oxford University Press; 2003.

47 General Medical Council. *Confidentiality: protecting and providing information.* London: General Medical Council; 2004.

CHAPTER 6

Cultural diversity and competence

This chapter explores:
- definitions of culture and competence
- teaching and learning cultural diversity
- racism in medicine
- culture shock.

> I think [that] in an understandable effort to get Australians to understand cultural diversity and pluralism, we've been reluctant to say that here are some values that are not negotiable. . . . We've been stuck on the debate about cultures, but we haven't discussed enough the values of those cultures.
>
> *John Roskam, Institute of Public Affairs, Melbourne, 2005*[1]

The above quote from John Roskam appeared in the Australian newspaper, *Weekend Australian*, a few months before ugly scenes of violence took place between gangs of youths on Sydney's southern beaches. The debate about multiculturalism and tolerance began in response to fears about religious and racial tension in the wake of the war in Iraq and the fear of 'militant clerics' preaching fundamentalism. Commentators on the beach riots, which appeared to be between white Australians and Australians of Lebanese descent, variously stated that the fighting between the two groups was and was not a sign of the inherent racism dormant in Australian society. In the UK there have been a number of high-profile incidents suggesting similar intolerance and racism – for example, the murder of teenager Stephen Lawrence in London in 1993. In the UK, a BBC Online survey in 2002 showed that more than half of those polled believed that they lived in a racist society, although they also stated that they thought Britain was less racist than it was 10 years ago.[2] This is the climate in which health professionals live and practise.

To state the obvious, we all live in a multicultural society. Health professionals themselves come from all nations, races and cultural backgrounds, and the patients with whom they interact are likewise from diverse backgrounds. Racism and prejudice have no place in such a society, while dealing differently with a patient or health worker on the basis of the colour of their skin, their religion or way they dress is not acceptable within any health service.

However, issues relating to cultural diversity have many layers. Cultural competence does not consist solely of knowing the beliefs of patients with regard to death, contraception or diet, for example. There is also a need to understand the arguments for and against multiculturalism, the differences in morbidity and mortality statistics between and within countries, and the ethical dimensions of working with patients whose moral and cultural values might be quite different from one's own.

How should a health professional behave if a patient's cultural values are at odds with the society in which he or she is working? Other questions that merit discussion relate to the tension between dealing with racism and working as an altruistic health professional. What is the professional way of dealing with racism against oneself or one's colleagues? Should or could a health professional refuse to help a patient who is making derogatory comments about the professional's colour or ethnicity?

SOME DEFINITIONS

Papers and discussion documents on this subject have been appearing with increasing frequency over the last decade. Health profession students are likely to encounter cultural diversity courses on their curriculum. These may be labelled as cultural competency, valuing diversity, cultural safety training or cultural awareness, to name just a few. Some of the definitions of such terms are shown in Box 6.1.

The ideal culturally safe and inclusive environment allows all people free speech and an expression of their point of view. However, within any society that upholds free speech, there may be exceptions to what is allowed. For example, in many countries it is unacceptable, and indeed often illegal, to incite violence, or to make racist or sexist comments. In certain countries where health professionals from democratic states choose to work, free speech may not be possible, women may not be able to talk with whomsoever they like, and not all ethnic groups are treated equally. Is 'valuing diversity' thus a Western construct? And even in the West do we truly value it?

BOX 6.1 DEFINITIONS RELATING TO CULTURAL DIVERSITY

Culture: The total way of life – the underlying pattern of thinking, feeling and acting – of particular groups of people.[3] How people make sense of their surroundings, including attitudes and behaviour, assumptions and values. What people 'take for granted', what they notice about others, but which is largely invisible to themselves.

Cultural awareness: Knowing and understanding that there are differences between people. Having insight into the physical, psychological, social, spiritual, economic and political context in which people live or have lived.

Cultural sensitivity: Insight into and reflection on how our own and others' culture affect our interactions and behaviour.

Cultural relativity: Understanding the cultural development of societies without trying to impose absolute moral ideals or trying to compare cultures against some form of absolute cultural standard.

Cultural competence: Competence itself has been defined as the ability to assume a combination of well-defined roles.[4] Cultural competency may therefore be defined as being able to give direct patient care to people from different cultural backgrounds.

Cultural intelligence: Engaging and balancing the head, heart and mind in new and/or uncomfortable cross-cultural situations.[5]

Cultural safety: An environment that is safe for people – where there is no challenge to, assault on or denial of their identity, of who they are and what they need. There is shared respect, shared meaning, shared knowledge and shared experience in addition to learning, living and working together with dignity and true listening.[6]

Culturally inclusive environment: In such an environment people from any cultural background can freely express who they are, give their own opinions and points of view, may fully participate in teaching, learning, work, social activities and healthcare, and can feel safe from abuse, harassment or unfair criticism.[7]

THE DIVERSITY WHEEL

Figure 6.1 shows one version of a diversity wheel[8] that brings together the various components of diversity that affect an individual and a society. The inner ring contains factors that we are born with or which we develop involuntarily. The outer ring represents factors that we can change or which are influenced by our environment, experience and upbringing, and about which we do have some choice. Ethnic heritage, race and religion are only a few of the influences that govern our health beliefs and attitudes.

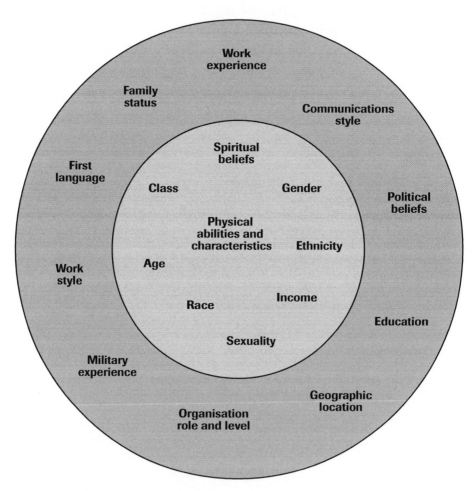

FIGURE 6.1 The diversity wheel.[8]

Race, ethnicity and culture are words that are often used synonymously. In particular, the terms 'racial group' and 'ethnic group' are interchangeable to many people. However, they in fact have different meanings. Race is defined primarily on physical grounds, ethnicity is psychological, and culture is socio-logical in broad terms.[9] Thus race is about physical appearance and genetic ancestry, and, although controversial, is deemed to be permanent. Culture relates to a person's behaviour and attitudes, is affected by upbringing and later choice, and can be changed. Group identity is an important component of ethnicity, and is determined by a sense of belonging as well as cultural ties and social forces.[9]

THE CULTURE OF THE MEDICAL PROFESSION

Apart from our own upbringing and cultural values relating to our society, health professionals are immersed in the culture of their own profession, with its health beliefs, language (jargon), rules of engagement and hierarchy. Topics discussed in this book are related to the cultural values of the profession – for example, the view that many doctors have that it is acceptable to self-diagnose and treat, and that doctors must stick together and regulate each other. Health professionals (in particular doctors) often 'talk shop' on social occasions and use black humour as a means of relieving stress and entertaining each other. Students entering training should discuss the culture in which they will work, understand its biases and values, and use this knowledge to help them to understand the cultures of the patients with whom they will interact.

REFLECTIONS ON TEACHING CULTURAL DIVERSITY

Cultural competency has been criticised as an attempt, while trying to ensure that medical students and doctors no longer hold ignorant or biased views about their patients, to reduce cultural issues to a simplistic level.[10] The 'cookbook approach' of lists of characteristics of different cultures, such as dietary taboos and funeral customs, presents them as static rather than dynamic. It is easy to stereotype, to attribute to one individual, the customs and attitudes of a whole group of people because of some similarities, bearing in mind that there are often as many differences *within* groups as there are between them. Education that focuses only on specific attributes and differences tends to distract students from reflecting on their attitudes and biases.[11]

As we know from our own backgrounds, whatever they may be, friends, relatives, working colleagues and acquaintances from the same 'cultural background' may hold very different opinions from our own and behave in contrasting ways. Two white female English-speaking 50-year-old patients living in the same street cannot be expected to have the same tastes in music and decoration, let alone the same ideas, concerns and expectations with regard to their health. Neither can two Asian male 35-year-old patients. If one of these patients is a highly trained professional and the other left school at 16 years of age and is unemployed, they will probably have quite different outlooks on life. One study of British Bangladeshi patients with diabetes found that their attitudes towards the condition were influenced not only by their cultural inheritance, but also by their social circumstances and level of deprivation – attributes that they shared with their non-Bangladeshi neighbours. The similarities were as striking as the differences in health beliefs between the two groups.[12] Cross-cultural education should therefore also address social factors, such as level of education, living standards, income, religion and support networks.[13]

Diversity involves not only cultural differences but also ethical and moral ones (*see* Chapter 3). Irvine and colleagues from the University of Newcastle, New South Wales, do not believe that contemporary biomedical ethics has 'adequately engaged with indigenous and non-Western ethical frameworks and modes of moral thought.'[14] To overcome this, professionals should be open to the cultures of others and recognise their own potential prejudices and assumptions. Cultural competency is now a requirement for US medical school accreditation, while the GMC is also asking about cultural diversity teaching on accreditation visits.

All health professionals should have the opportunity to attend cultural diversity training, to discuss both generic competencies and those specific to the patient groups with whom they work. In Australia, for example, cultural safety training is directed mainly at promoting an understanding of the Aboriginal and Torres Strait Islander population, but will also focus on the Indigenous groups of the area. Such training is carried out not only by a clinical educator but also by a cultural mentor of Indigenous background. Storytellers from the local communities share the narrative of their lives, which are a rich resource for all participants. Learning about one culture in depth should open up cultural perspectives and reduce provincialism – 'by helping one to see more clearly the characteristics of one's own society and culture and heightening one's appreciation of commonalities and differences among cultures.'[15]

Topics for discussion at cultural diversity/safety workshops are suggested in Box 6.2, and these will be tailored to local needs. These learning experiences are best run as interactive sessions. Participants should be able to challenge each other if unhelpful or harmful statements are made. It is important to establish ground rules at the beginning of the sessions.

BOX 6.2 IDEAS FOR DISCUSSION AT DIVERSITY WORKSHOPS

- Definitions (as above in Box 6.1).
- Discussion of one's own culture and what this means.
- How to be culturally aware and provide a culturally safe environment for professionals and patients.
- Communication and potential problems.
- Possible differences in health beliefs and world views between cultural groups, and how these might affect the accessing of healthcare.
- Gender differences and how these might affect professional–patient interactions.
- Family structure and dynamics and their bearing on healthcare.
- Confidentiality: does this differ?
- Treatment of children and the elderly.
- Attitudes to medicine taking and modes of delivery.

With regard to specific groups, health professionals should be aware of common beliefs, with an understanding that these should be checked, as they cannot be assumed for any individual. Knowledge of dietary restrictions, customs with regard to birth and death, and traditional medical practices is important. However, professional behaviour is such that if a health worker does not know, he or she should ask in a polite way. The professional should also ensure that the patient understands what is happening.

From a purely biomedical perspective, clinicians must be aware of differences between racial groups with regard to incidence of disease, risk factors and differences in the effects of drugs. From an ethical perspective, this means that there will be differences between such groups with regard to interventions. In the UK, the National Institute for Health and Clinical Excellence (NICE), in its document on social value judgements, states in Principle 9 that 'NICE clinical guidance should only recommend the use of an intervention for a particular racial (ethnic) group if there is clear evidence of differences between racial (ethnic) groups in the clinical effectiveness of the intervention that cannot be identified by any other means.'[16]

EXPLORING HEALTH BELIEFS IN A CULTURALLY SENSITIVE WAY

The patient-centred approach to consultations is an appropriate method of interaction when there are cultural and/or ethnic differences between patient and health professional. Exploring a patient's ideas, concerns and expectations is important in any consultation, and this model translates well when the aim is to provide culturally competent healthcare. Language may also be a barrier, and an interpreter may be required (*see* Chapter 5 for further details). However, if language is not seen to be a problem, a patient's ideas and concerns may appear very different from those of one's own background.

Health professionals who have been trained in the Western biomedical tradition may be used to 'old wives' tales' regarding diagnosis and treatment, as they have probably been exposed to such beliefs from childhood. However, when interacting with patients from other medical traditions, many of their explanations for illness and disease may seem very strange. The health professional may try to apply the patient-centred model and begin to explore the patient's ideas, but this may not be successful if the patient is from a culture in which the doctor is regarded as a figure of authority, who is not to be questioned. Some patients may expect a paternalistic healer and be unprepared for sharing decisions and/or choosing options. Box 6.3 lists some of the areas that health professionals should explore with patients. One useful question is 'What methods or tools can I, as your health provider, use to help you learn more about your current illness or surgery?'[17]

BOX 6.3 AREAS TO EXPLORE IN CONSULTATIONS

- What the patient identifies as his or her cultural group.
- Length of time in this country (whether born here or immigrated).
- Previous experiences of medical treatment in home country/host country.
- Use of 'traditional' medicines or alternative medical practices.
- Spiritual beliefs and how these may impact on illness.
- Who else is involved in making decisions about healthcare (e.g. family, priest, religious mentor).
- The meaning of this illness to the patient.
- Health beliefs.

In the field of mental health there are many pitfalls to consider when interacting with patients from cultures outside the Western view of mental illness. Health professionals are commonly used to working within the classification system of the Western tradition, namely the *Diagnostic and Statistical Manual of Mental Disorders (DSM-IV)*. Although a number of cultural features have been incorporated into the DSM-IV, particularly in the glossary of 'culture-bound syndromes', there are still problems with cultural fallacies, in which the diagnostic categories of one culture are applied to patients from another culture.[18] Again, unless the ideas and concerns of the patient (and their family) are explored, a full picture of the problem will not be forthcoming, and treatment is likely to fail due to non-adherence. Health professionals need to consider non-Western theories of illness causation – for example, fate, the evil eye, spirit possession, powerful dreams, violation of a taboo or coming into contact with an unclean object (e.g. a dead body).[18]

WORKING IN A MULTICULTURAL HEALTH SERVICE

Leininger, the founder of the transcultural nursing movement in the USA, has described three possible modes of healthcare intervention.[19] The first mode, *care oriented towards cultural preservation*, involves acknowledging a patient's cultural health beliefs and working with them in a complementary way with one's own 'orthodox' views. The second mode, *cultural negotiation*, involves each party trying to understand the other's viewpoint and compromise where necessary to ensure the best outcome for the patient. The third mode, *cultural repatterning*, is more controversial, as it involves the health professional challenging the patient's way of life because it is unacceptable in the society in which the health professional is living and practising. Look again at the quote at the beginning of this chapter. Discussion about cultural tolerance has been high on the agenda following terrorist activities during 2005.

On careful reflection it should be obvious what falls outside culturally acceptable practice in the country in which we are working. Practice that is not acceptable on this basis is often illegal. In the UK, an example of this is doctors refusing to perform female circumcision (female genital mutilation). This operation is now illegal in the UK, although it may be requested by certain groups. However, professionalism, with its inherent code of conduct, means that we must continually challenge ourselves, and any attempt at 'repatterning' must be subjected to close scrutiny. A key question we need to ask ourselves is in whose interests we are acting.

Western medicine's moves toward patient autonomy and shared decision making may not be the best framework within which to interact with patients from some cultural backgrounds. For example, health professionals in the UK have a strict code of confidentiality. However, some patients may expect test results to be given to the head of the family, or a decision on treatment to be made by an elder. It is important to establish precisely what forms of communication will be used between patient, family and health professional.

A PROFESSIONAL APPROACH TO RACISM

Health professionals are likely to be confronted by racism fairly often in their daily activities. Sometimes the racism may be fairly subtle. For example, a patient whose GP wants to refer him to a specialist may ask for a referral to a British doctor (the subtext being 'white' doctor). Is this different from a patient with limited English asking to see a doctor who speaks Punjabi? In the latter case the doctor could be from anywhere in the world and be of any ethnic background – it is the language that is the important factor. Or is it? Is that what the patient is really asking for?

Should we try to accommodate patients who wish to see doctors of a particular ethnic or racial background? How should we respond to the request of the first patient? Should we ignore the underlying message and refer them to the 'best' doctor (or indeed the only doctor) available?

Racial prejudice and racism are related concepts with subtle differences in meaning. Racial prejudice arises from attitudes and beliefs, is often based on misperception and ignorance, and may be caused by insecurity.[9] Racism is an ideological and political stance, arising from assumptions about inferior and superior races, with undertones of power and domination. It may be the result of social conditioning and history.[9] Thus racial prejudice is the feeling and racism is the behaviour.

The Macpherson Report into the murder of teenager Stephen Lawrence included a definition of institutional racism as 'the collective failure of an organisation to provide an appropriate and professional service to people because of their colour, culture or ethnic origin. It can be seen or detected in processes, attitudes and behaviour which amount to discrimination through unwitting prejudice, ignorance, thoughtlessness and racist stereotyping which disadvantages minority ethnic people.'[20] Racism in society 'acts as a major hurdle to health and wealth.'[20] To avoid racism in the health service (which is still widespread[21]), patients should be involved in professional development. Health professionals should discuss the cases described above and decide on the best ways to tackle them, with a skilled facilitator to ensure that all of the options are considered and all of the participants feel that it is safe for them to contribute. Any service or institution that provides healthcare needs a policy for dealing with racist remarks made both by staff and towards staff.

One study from an educational setting has shown that the strongest unique predictor of a person's attitude to people from different cultural or 'foreign' backgrounds is whether there is difficulty in communication. This difficulty could arise from accented speech, inability to speak each other's language, or differences in non-verbal communication. Lack of communication then causes discomfort, impatience and frustration, leading to prejudice.[22] Chapter

5 discusses the use of interpreters to overcome some of these communication barriers.

CULTURE SHOCK

When people move to a new job, a new school, a new city or a new country, after an initial period of anticipation and euphoria they may often become unhappy or uncomfortable. The experience of change from familiar surroundings, customs, ways of working and timetables, leading to anxiety, is known as 'culture shock.' Recognition of culture shock and having the means to work through it oneself or to help others, including peers, patients and students, are key professional skills. Health professionals who come into contact with patients and students deal with the effects of culture shock on a regular basis. They also experience the phenomenon themselves when they move hospitals, when they move into primary care from a secondary care setting and vice versa, and when they change bosses, become promoted, or undertake postgraduate study.

Culture shock can affect a person's emotions, behaviour and physical health. Uncertainty and bewilderment usually settle within three to six months if the person adapts to the change in circumstances. Box 6.4 shows ways in which colleagues, friends or the institution may respond and help to deal with culture shock, as well as what an individual may do to help him- or herself.

BOX 6.4 WAYS TO OVERCOME CULTURE SHOCK

- Be welcoming.
- Take time to get to know new people.
- Organise social events (check diet and drink prohibitions first).
- Attend social events.
- Smile.
- Hold orientation sessions for new people.
- Ensure that support mechanisms are in place and that people know how to access them.
- Maintain contact with old friends and family.
- Exercise, as this helps to reduce stress.
- Give details on how to register with a local GP.
- Register with a GP.

SUMMARY

Although definitions of professionalism include altruism and specialist knowledge, there has often not been an explicit discussion of the competencies required for professionals to interact with people from different cultures. Courses in cultural diversity, or courses with similar names to this, are now included in both undergraduate and postgraduate training, but they vary in content and focus. Health professionals not only need to be able to work without discrimination, but they also need to be able to work within an environment where they themselves may be subject to discrimination and/ or racism.

REFERENCES

1 Eccleston R, Legge K. Cracks in the Melting Pot. *Weekend Australian*, 23–24 July 2005, p. 19.
2 http://news.bbc.co.uk/1/hi/uk/1993597.stm (accessed May 2008).
3 O'Hara-Devereaux M, Johansen R. *Global Work: bridging distance, culture and time.* San Francisco, CA: Jossey-Bass; 1994.
4 Schuwirth LWT, van der Vleuten CPM. Changing education, changing assessment, changing research. *Med Educ.* 2004; **38**: 805–12.
5 Earley C, Ang S. *Cultural Intelligence: individual interactions across cultures.* Palo Alto, CA: Stanford University Press; 2003.
6 Williams R. *Working in a Culturally Safe Environment;* www.flinders.edu.au/kokotinna/SECT04/OVERVW.htm (accessed July 2005).
7 Flinders University. *Cultural Diversity and Inclusive Practice Toolkit;* www.flinders.au/equal-opportunity/cdip/ (accessed May 2008).
8 Loden M. *Implementing Diversity.* Chicago, IL: Irwin Professional Publishing; www.loden.com/Site/Dimensions.html (accessed March 2008).
9 Fernando S. *Mental Health, Race and Culture.* 2nd ed. Basingstoke: Palgrave; 2002.
10 Wear D. Insurgent multiculturalism: rethinking how and why we teach culture in medical education. *Acad Med.* 2003; **78**: 549–54.
11 Kai J, Bridgwater R, Spencer J. '"Just think of TB and Asians", that's all I ever hear': medical learners' views about training to work in an ethnically diverse society. *Med Educ.* 2001; **35**: 250–56.
12 Greenhalgh T, Helman C, Chowdhury M. Health beliefs and folk models of diabetes in British Bangladeshis: a qualitative study. *BMJ.* 1998; **316**: 978–83.
13 Green AR, Betancourt JR, Carrillo JE. Integrating social factors into cross-cultural medical education. *Acad Med.* 2002; **77**: 193–7.
14 Irvine R, McPhee J, Kerridge IH. The challenge of cultural and ethical pluralism to medical practice. *Med J Aust.* 2002; **176**: 174–5.
15 Fox RC. Cultural competence and the culture of medicine. *NEJM.* 2005; **353**: 1316–19.
16 National Institute for Health and Clinical Excellence (NICE). *Social Value Judgements. Principles for the development of NICE guidelines;* www.nice.org.uk/pdf/SocialValueJudgement-08_12_05.pdf (accessed January 2006).

17 Joint Commission Resources. *Providing Culturally and Linguistically Competent Health Care*. Chicago, IL: Joint Commission Resources; 2006.

18 Andary L, Stolk Y, Klimidis S. *Assessing Mental Health Across Cultures*. Bowen Hills, Queensland: Australian Academic Press; 2003.

19 Leininger MM. Cultural care diversity and universality. *Nurs Sci Q*. 1988; **1**: 152–60.

20 Macpherson W. *The Stephen Lawrence Inquiry Report*. London: The Stationery Office; 1999.

21 Gould M. Report accuses NHS of institutional racism. *BMJ*. 2004; **328**: 367.

22 Spencer-Rodgers J, McGovern T. Attitudes toward the culturally different: the role of intercultural communication barriers, affective responses, consensual stereotypes and perceived threat. *Int J Intercult Relat*. 2002; **26**: 609–31.

CHAPTER 7

Professional knowledge and development: keeping up to date

This chapter explores:
- the nature of professional knowledge
- keeping up to date
- continuing professional development
- assessing learning needs
- competence and performance
- demonstrating competence
- evidence-based practice
- work-based learning.

> Doctors must be committed to lifelong learning and be responsible for maintaining the medical knowledge and clinical and team skills necessary for the provision of quality care.
>
> *Medical Professionalism Project, 2002*[1]

> It [the Senate of Surgery's response to the events in Bristol] also warned that political projects such as waiting-list initiatives put patient safety at risk. They put undue pressure on doctors and prevented them from keeping up to date with training, it said.
>
> *The BBC Online network, 1998*[2]

As we have already seen, one of the hallmarks of a profession is the presence of skill based on specialist knowledge. In the case of medicine, these skills and knowledge are first learned at medical school. Specialisation occurs after graduation, with further knowledge and skills being learned 'on the job', both through experience and from role models (the apprenticeship model), formal teaching courses and reading of the biomedical literature. The aspiring specialist then sits one or more professional examinations and, unless they choose voluntarily to undertake a further degree or diploma, the successful doctor no longer has to study formally for any further assessments.

However, doctors are expected to keep up to date within their field through continuing professional development and appraisal. One of the prime professional attributes that medical graduates are expected to acquire during their long and arduous education is the desire for *lifelong learning*. They also need the tools to carry this out, including critical appraisal, as not everything that is published will have an impact on one's work (or even be true).

A more formal process of revalidation may include clinical examinations or the results of other methods of demonstrating continuing quality performance. However, we must ask how successful health professionals are at keeping abreast of professional knowledge in this era of information overload, accelerating medical discoveries and ever increasing work pressure. And what effect does this have on professionalism, with its emphasis on technical knowledge and skills?

THE NATURE OF PROFESSIONAL KNOWLEDGE

Michael Eraut, Professor of Education at the University of Sussex, has written a great deal on the nature and acquisition of professional knowledge. This unique profession-specific knowledge and expertise confers power and status on professionals. The less accessible and more unintelligible the knowledge is to lay people, the greater the power imbalance. Eraut suggests that professions prefer to present this knowledge base as:

➤ carrying the aura of uncertainty associated with established scientific disciplines

➤ sufficiently erudite to justify a long period of training, preferably to degree level for all, with specialist postgraduate training beyond that for some

➤ different from that of all other occupations.[3]

Of course the health professions can now only be entered via a university degree, and all doctors undergo specialist training of some kind. Schön defined the knowledge base of a profession as having four essential properties: 'It is specialised, firmly bounded, scientific and standardised.'[4]

Although all health professionals learn their profession-specific generic knowledge, the influence of personal experiences, caseload, the 'hidden curriculum' and role models leads to a personal knowledge base that varies from one individual to another. Eraut defines this distinction as the difference between 'propositional knowledge' (that underpinning or enabling professional action, the knowledge taught explicitly at university and found in textbooks) and 'practical know-how.' As Eraut points out, this mirrors what Aristotle described as 'technical knowledge' and 'practical knowledge.'[3] Tacit knowledge is defined as what professionals know but cannot describe.[5] How do we explain to students the way that we often rely on intuition or professional judgement and 'just know' that something is the case? The works of Schön highlight the importance of reflection for the assimilation of new knowledge and translating knowledge into practice.[4] Professional 'judgement involves practical wisdom, a sense of purpose, appropriateness and feasibility; and its acquisition depends, among other things, on a wealth of professional experience.'[3]

YOUTH VERSUS EXPERIENCE

Clinical tutors find themselves in an unusual position with regard to students of the health professions. On the one hand, the tutors can draw upon their wide-ranging clinical experience, personal patient databases and multiple illness narratives in their teaching. On the other hand, senior students are more likely than their tutors to know of recent developments in biomedical sciences and pharmacology. One of the incentives for many doctors, particularly GPs, during medical students' clinical attachments is that the doctors often learn as much as the students, and in addition the teaching inspires them to keep up to date.[6]

It would seem logical that senior clinicians with their greater experience provide better patient care than their more junior colleagues. However, this depends on what we mean by patient care. Two American doctors conducted a systematic review in 2005 which demonstrated that older doctors have less factual knowledge, are less likely to follow appropriate standards of care, and have poorer patient outcomes than younger practitioners. Overall, they found a negative association between the number of years a doctor had been in practice and the quality of their performance.[7]

What are the implications of these findings? Can an older health professional improve their standard of care by appropriate education, or do we have to accept that the ageing brain and loss of manual dexterity over time may compromise patient care? There must be a point at which a doctor changes from becoming more proficient to becoming less so. This raises the question of how long a doctor should practise. There is probably no one age limit that is suitable for all. The mandatory retirement age for doctors in the UK is 70 years, although many retire before this through choice. Once revalidation is introduced, some doctors may be forced to retire even though they do not want to do so. Others may be recommended to change what they do. For example, surgeons may be advised not to operate but only to see outpatients.

As well as considering at what point a professional should retire from practice, the other question that relates to professional knowledge and skills is how much clinical work is enough to enable one to continue to practise at the highest level that one can. This is particularly important as many health professionals now work part-time. Some combine their clinical work with raising families, while others combine it with other types of work, such as teaching, research and management. Knowledge and skills atrophy if they are not used regularly. Is one day a week of clinical work enough? One attribute of professionalism, then, should be the ability to know when to stop practising as a clinician or to restrict one's practice in line with one's knowledge and skills.

CONTINUING PROFESSIONAL DEVELOPMENT

The health professions expect their members to keep up to date and to provide evidence of continuing professional development (CPD). In the past, continuing medical education (CME) was the term with regard to doctors. CPD recognises that development includes learning not only about the clinical aspects of one's job, but also about team working, management and teaching. CPD thus offers a broader range of professional enhancement. Overall, in the short term CPD should help practitioners to maintain and improve their knowledge and skills, while also providing opportunities for them to learn new knowledge and skills. In the long term this should translate into improved performance, better patient care and better patient outcomes. Box 7.1 gives the Academy of Royal Medical Colleges' definition of CPD. In the UK the Royal Colleges are responsible for providing a framework for continuing professional development, setting educational standards, and monitoring, facilitating and evaluating activities for their members.

BOX 7.1 DEFINITION OF CPD[8]

Continuing professional development is a process of lifelong learning for all individuals and teams which enables them to meet the needs of patients and to deliver the healthcare priorities of the National Health Service and other employers, and which enables professionals to expand and fulfil their potential.

Health professionals who attend CPD-accredited courses or participate in other accredited activities, such as distance learning or e-learning packages, receive credits for such participation. However, credits are only counted, and little attention is paid to what the professional actually learned. Although ideally a health professional should undertake education to improve patient care, internationally there are a variety of incentives on offer to entice the reluctant professional to participate. These include financial rewards or penalties, mandatory contracts with health insurers, being on the publicised list of accredited specialists, and continuing registration to practise.[9]

BOX 7.2 CHARACTERISTICS OF USEFUL CPD ACTIVITIES

- Formulation of an individual learning plan.
- Activities should be balanced, varied, and not focused on only one area or topic.
- Regular.
- Should not concentrate on what is known or what is liked. Move out of the 'comfort zone.'
- Should include evidence of learning.
- Should include a reflective element.
- May be related to audit activity.

The dedicated professional does not just turn up to be lectured to, to be given handouts that are never read, or to leave an event early once he has been signed in for the session. The dedicated professional, as an adult learner, plans their CPD. Box 7.2 includes the characteristics that should be considered when planning or undertaking CPD during one's career. Only attending educational sessions that focus on organisational change, departmental planning, career development or new breakthroughs is not a balanced approach. CPD needs to include elements that improve the quality of one's existing performance. As Eraut warns, 'the potential of work-related, if not always work-based, mid-career professional education is underestimated. Instead of helping professionals to reformulate their theories of practice in the light of their semi-digested case experiences and under the stimulus of collegial sharing and challenging, CPE (continuing professional education) all too often provides yet another strand of separate, unintegrated and therefore minimally used, professional knowledge.'[3]

COMPETENCE AND PERFORMANCE

When discussing a health professional's ability to practise, we often use the words 'competence' and 'performance' interchangeably. However, the education literature distinguishes between the two (*see* Box 7.3), and this becomes important when considering the assessment of poorly performing doctors. Competence is assessed by staged examinations, such as consultations with simulated patients or observation of doctors' clinical skills on mannequins. Assessment of performance requires work-based observation and is thus less feasible, prone to be less reliable, and likely to interfere with the smooth running of the clinical environment. A professional may demonstrate competence in an assessment, but may not always perform well in the workplace. Continuing professional development should aim to enhance performance, and thus the success of CPD is difficult to assess. As Eraut wrote, 'Proficiency on routine is essential for competence, but it is the handling of non-routine matters which is responsible for excellence.'[3] Perhaps we could substitute 'performance' for 'excellence' in that statement.

BOX 7.3 COMPETENCE AND PERFORMANCE

Competence: The ability to do the job. What doctors do in controlled representations of professional practice.[10]

Performance: The ability to do the job well. What doctors do in their professional practice.[10]

PERSONAL DEVELOPMENT PLANS

CPD comes with its own jargon. One way of documenting learning needs and the activities undertaken to meet those needs is the personal development plan (PDP) – a learning plan with a diary of activity. When evidence of learning with reflection is added to this, the PDP becomes a portfolio. A portfolio in medical education is a collection of documents (or other materials) providing such evidence of learning and a reflective account of those documented events.[11] The evidence shows that the stated objectives or outcomes of the educational activity have been achieved. Furthermore, a portfolio should demonstrate that the professional has reached the required standard for their level of training or practice. This standard includes fitness to practise and the right professional attributes. It is likely that revalidation will involve some form of portfolio-based assessment when it is finally introduced.

When designing a PDP, the professional has to decide on their learning needs or educational priorities. Rughani has identified eight questions to be answered when setting an educational priority[12] (*see* Box 7.4). The crucial elements are what needs to be learned, how one knows one needs to learn it and, to close the loop, how one knows that one has learned it. Without evidence of learning, the plan will be incomplete. Junior health professionals may either feel that they need to learn too much, and therefore their plans become unwieldy and overwhelming, or that they in fact don't know what they don't know. Therefore they will need guidance from clinical tutors. Good advice is to select just three educational priorities or learning objectives at a time. Trigger questions for setting objectives are suggested in Box 7.5.

BOX 7.4 QUESTIONS TO BE ANSWERED WITH REGARD TO PDPs

- What is the general area in which I need to learn?
- How have I established this need?
- What is the aim of my learning?
- What are the specific objectives that I wish to achieve?
- How do I intend to achieve these objectives?
- How will I evaluate my development plan?
- How will I demonstrate that I have undertaken this plan?
- What is my timescale?

BOX 7.5 TRIGGER QUESTIONS FOR ESTABLISHING LEARNING NEEDS

Considering the patients I am about to consult with or am about to admit:
- What three conditions would I least like to have to deal with?
- Which type of patients would I be least comfortable with?
- What do I hope I do not have to do today?

Considering the patients who have consulted me today or whom I have seen on the wards:

- Which do I feel least happy about?
- Were there any conditions I was unable to manage?
- What drugs was I unsure about (side-effects, dosage, interaction)?
- What areas of my clinical practice do I feel are getting out of date?
- What skills do I need to acquire or improve?
- What critical incidents have occurred during my practice this week?

Trigger questions and other sources of information that feed into a learning plan are the basis of an individual's 'educational needs assessment.' Such needs assessments may also be carried out by institutions, often following a critical incident or adverse report.

Professor Janet Grant of the Open University and her colleagues have identified many such sources of information to help with educational planning, and have collated them into *The Good CPD Guide*.[13] Professor Grant has also classified seven different types of needs assessment from which to choose when planning CPD (*see* Box 7.6).

BOX 7.6 METHODS OF EDUCATIONAL NEEDS ASSESSMENT[14]

- *Gap or discrepancy analysis:* This formal method involves comparing performance with stated intended competencies – by self-assessment, peer assessment or objective testing – and planning education accordingly.
- *Reflection-on-action and reflection-in-action:* Reflection-on-action is an aspect of experiential learning and involves thinking back to some performance, with or without triggers (e.g. videotape or audiotape), and identifying what was done well and what could have been done better.
- *Self-assessment by diaries, journals, log books or weekly reviews:* This is an extension of reflection that involves keeping a diary or other account of experiences.
- *Peer review:* This involves doctors assessing each other's practice and giving feedback and perhaps advice about possible education, training or organisational strategies to improve performance.
- *Observation:* Doctors can be observed performing specific tasks that can be rated by an observer, either according to known criteria or more informally. The results are discussed, and learning needs are identified.
- *Critical incident review and significant event auditing:* Although this

technique is usually used to identify the competencies of a profession or for quality assurance, it can also be used on an individual basis to identify learning needs. The method involves individuals identifying and recording, say, one incident each week in which they feel they should have performed better, analysing the incident according to its setting, exactly what occurred, and the outcome and why it was ineffective.

- *Practice review:* A routine review of notes, charts, prescribing, letters, requests, etc. can identify learning needs, especially if the format of looking at what is satisfactory and what leaves room for improvement is followed.

EVIDENCE OF LEARNING

Students are used to being assessed formally to provide evidence of learning. Postgraduates also have examinations, but their performance is also scrutinised by their seniors and their peers. True adult learners who feel that their continuing professional development relates to their wanting to improve themselves and do better for patients will have other means of providing evidence. Evidence is thus of two kinds – proof to me that I have learned something, and proof to an outside person that learning has taken place. The second kind is the basis of assessment and revalidation. Evidence may come in various forms, including examination results (*see* Box 7.7). We can put all of this together in the evidence cycle (*see* Figure 7.1).

BOX 7.7 TYPES OF EVIDENCE

- Audit of skills activity which shows improvement in outcomes.
- List of patients seen with the conditions on my learning plan, and outcomes for these. Did I deal with them more successfully? How do I know this?
- Reflection on learning.
- Data to show that more patients are coming back to see me with certain conditions.
- Prescription data.
- 360-degree appraisal forms.
- References from previous posts.
- Certificates of attendance at educational meetings (with reflection on what has been learned).
- Diplomas or higher degrees obtained.
- Published papers.

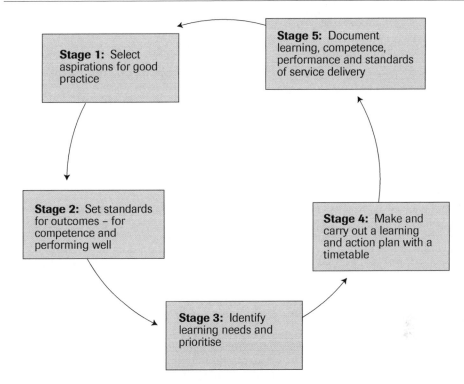

FIGURE 7.1 Evidence cycle (adapted from Chambers *et al.*[15]).

EVIDENCE-BASED MEDICINE

So far we have been considering the process of CPD and the ways for an individual professional to decide on its content. In broad terms what should be the content in order to keep up to date with medical advances? The evidence-based medicine (EBM) or evidence-based practice movement suggests that all clinical work should have evidence to support it, and thus the professional needs to keep abreast of such evidence and its shifts.

Evidence-based medicine (EBM) can be defined as:

> . . . the conscientious, explicit, and judicious use of current best evidence in making decisions about the care of individual patients. The practice of evidence-based medicine means integrating individual clinical expertise with the best available external clinical evidence from systematic research. By individual clinical expertise we mean the proficiency and judgment that individual clinicians acquire through clinical experience and clinical practice. Increased expertise is reflected in many ways, but especially in more effective and efficient diagnosis and in the more thoughtful identification and compassionate use of

individual patients' predicaments, rights, and preferences in making clinical decisions about their care. By best available external clinical evidence we mean clinically relevant research, often from the basic sciences of medicine, but especially from patient-centred clinical research into the accuracy and precision of diagnostic tests (including the clinical examination), the power of prognostic markers, and the efficacy and safety of therapeutic, rehabilitative, and preventive regimens. External clinical evidence both invalidates previously accepted diagnostic tests and treatments and replaces them with new ones that are more powerful, more accurate, more efficacious, and safer.[16]

Doctors may be praised or damned by being described as 'old-fashioned.' Some patients may relate this description to their doctor being courteous, paternalistic and understanding of their family circumstances and history. The old-fashioned doctor makes house calls and soothes the fevered brows of his patients – the personal touch. Other people see old-fashioned doctors as out of date, persisting in using remedies that may have no objective evidence to suggest that they work, or, if such medication is efficacious, it has been superseded by newer and more effective drugs.

Within the EBM paradigm all investigations and management should be evidence based. The practitioner asks questions in order to decide on the best treatment plan, looks for the evidence, weighs it up (hopefully involving the patient in the decision-making process) and follows through (*see* Box 7.8).

BOX 7.8 STEPS INVOLVED IN EVIDENCE-BASED MEDICINE[17]

---

1 Convert information needs into answerable questions.
2 Track down the best evidence to answer these questions.
3 Critically appraise the evidence for its validity and importance.
4 Integrate this appraisal with clinical expertise and patient values to apply the results in clinical practice.
5 Evaluate performance.

PROBLEMS WITH ADOPTING AN EVIDENCE-BASED APPROACH

A major problem with clinical work is the speed with which advances are being made in medicine. Clinicians are often confronted by questions that cannot be answered on the spot. These may form the basis for this month's learning plan, but what should be done if the patient's management requires an answer now? Doctors need to have the knowledge and skills to search for evidence when faced with unusual presentations. They also need to be able to evaluate information that patients provide – perhaps data that they have accessed on the Internet or read about in the media. The busy clinician in the middle of an overbooked morning surgery is unlikely to find the time to search for the answer to a clinical question. Providing as much synthesised information as possible, that is easily accessible, at the doctor's desk is absolutely essential for EBM to translate into practice.

Such knowledge translation is defined as the exchange, synthesis and ethically sound application of knowledge, within a complex system of inter-actions among researchers and users, to accelerate the capture of the benefits of research – in other words, putting the results of research into practice.[18] In order to do this, professionals need to be able to cope with change, and the right conditions must be present in their practice and within the health services.

Doctors may try to adopt the EBM approach, but they also use the evidence of their own clinical 'trials' to decide on management. The trial of one method is a common reason to choose treatment. If a doctor prescribes a new drug for the first time and the patient has an adverse reaction to it, the doctor, despite published evidence with regard to the safety profile of the drug, is unlikely to prescribe that drug again, especially if there are alternatives that can be offered. This trial of one method is consistent with the theory that doctors make diagnostic and treatment decisions based on the 'illness scripts' of patients whom they have seen in the past.[19]

Gabbay and le May from the University of Southampton have described the collectively reinforced and internalised tacit guidelines that doctors use in everyday practice as 'mindlines.' They include brief reading, interactions with peers, opinion leaders, patients and pharmaceutical representatives, as well as their early training and their own experience.[20] As already mentioned above, the word 'tacit' refers to 'knowledge in practice', the informal process of experiential learning involving reflection, in contrast to explicit knowledge derived from research.

INFORMATION OVERLOAD

There are 2000 articles published each week in 20 000 biomedical journals. Reduce this number to those that are specifically about one's area of practice and there is still a lot of reading to fit into the busy working day. Moreover, within the medical press there is a bias towards publishing positive results.[21] However, this situation is likely to change following a directive from the editors of medical journals that all clinical trials must be registered so that both negative and positive results are in the public domain.[22] Such a standpoint should help doctors in their professional judgements.

Another way to overcome possible bias is for clinicians to read *systematic reviews*. These reviews help busy professionals to assess evidence by presenting, criticising and formulating as much of the published evidence as possible on a particular topic. Systematic reviews are scientific investigations (quantitative or qualitative) that include a synthesis of the results of multiple primary investigations by using strategies that limit bias and random error.[23] Meta-analyses are quantitative reviews that use statistical methods to combine the results of two or more studies. Qualitative reviews summarise primary studies without statistically combining them.[21]

SYSTEMATIC REVIEWS: THE COCHRANE COLLABORATION

The Cochrane Collaboration is an international organisation established in 1993 that sifts medical evidence in order to produce systematic reviews across all specialties.[24] The work is carried out by around 11 000 health professionals, researchers, scientists and consumers. Cochrane Reviews set out to answer clearly formulated questions of the type that clinicians ask every day in the course of their work. They are therefore an important resource for those who wish to update their medical knowledge and base this on firm evidence.

WORK-BASED LEARNING AND REFLECTION

Systematic reviews and other journal articles help practitioners to acquire new knowledge, but professionals do most of their learning 'on the job' through practical experience. They also learn from people. Clinicians consult with a large number of patients every year, and hopefully are learning something from each case. The doctor may not need to look up formally what a particular patient's constellation of symptoms and signs signifies, or research into the optimum treatment, but each doctor–patient interaction provides an opportunity to learn something new – about the human condition, communication, how illness progresses differently, health beliefs, etc. This knowledge is assimilated almost subconsciously, but professional development from such work-based learning only occurs if there is reflection on the events. Such learning occurring in the context of the daily workplace is far more likely to be relevant and reinforced, leading to better practice.[25]

SUMMARY

The public expects health professionals to be up to date in their clinical knowledge and expertise, although patients are prepared to accept that not all professionals are specialists in every field. A professional response to being asked about something that one does not know is to admit this and promise to find out, or refer the patient to someone else. Professionals should know the limits of their own knowledge and skills, and when to stop working if they cannot keep these up to an acceptable standard. Health professionals will have to demonstrate both competence and performance in the future in order to be able to carry on practising.

REFERENCES

1 Medical Professionalism Project. Medical professionalism in the new millennium: a physicians' charter. *Lancet*. 2002; **359**: 520–22.
2 http://news.bbc.co.uk/1/hi/health/background_briefings/the_bristol_heart_babies/198740.stm (accessed May 2008).
3 Eraut M. *Developing Professional Knowledge and Competence*. London: Routledge Falmer; 1994.
4 Schön DA. *Educating the Reflective Practitioner: towards a new design for teaching and learning in the professions*. San Francisco, CA: Jossey-Bass; 1987.
5 Polanyi M. *The Tacit Dimension*. London: Routledge; 1967.
6 Thistlethwaite JE, Storr E. The views of general practitioner tutors on developing medical students' communication and management skills. *Educ Primary Care*. 2004; **15**: 372–9.
7 Choudhry NK, Fletcher RH, Soumerai ScD. Systematic review: the relationship between clinical experience and quality of health care. *Ann Intern Med*. 2005; **142**: 260–73.
8 Academy of the Royal Medical Colleges. *A Framework for CPD Systems*. London: Academy of the Royal Medical Colleges; 1998.
9 Peck C, McCall M, McLaren B *et al*. Continuing medical education and continuing professional development: international comparisons. *BMJ*. 2000; **320**: 432–5.
10 Rethans J-J, Norcini JJ, Baron-Maldonado M *et al*. The relationship between competence and performance: implications for assessing practice performance. *Med Educ*. 2002; **36**: 901–9.
11 Snadden D, Thomas ML. The use of portfolio learning in medical education. *Med Teacher*. 1998; **20**: 192–9.
12 Rughani A. *The GP's Guide to Personal Development Plans*. 2nd ed. Oxford: Radcliffe Medical Press; 2001.
13 Grant J, Chambers G, Jackson G, editors. *The Good CPD Guide*. Sutton: Reed Healthcare; 1999.
14 Grant J. Learning needs assessment: assessing the need. *BMJ*. 2002; **324**: 156–9.
15 Chambers R, Mohanna K, Wakley G *et al*. *Demonstrating Your Competence. 1. Healthcare Teaching*. Oxford: Radcliffe Publishing; 2004.

16 Sackett DL, Rosenberg WMC, Muir Gray JA *et al.* Evidence-based medicine: what it is and what it isn't. *BMJ.* 1996; **312**: 71–2.

17 Straus SE, McAllister FA. Evidence-based medicine: a commentary on common criticisms. *Can Med Assoc J.* 2000; **163**: 837–41.

18 Davis D, Evans M, Jadad A *et al.* The case for knowledge translation: shortening the journey from evidence to effect. *BMJ.* 2003; **327**: 33–5.

19 Schmidt HG, Norman GR, Boshuizen HPA. A cognitive perspective on medical expertise: theory and implications. *Acad Med.* 1990; **65**: 611–21.

20 Gabbay, J, le May A. Evidence-based guidelines or collectively constructed 'mindlines'? Ethnographic study of knowledge management in primary care. *BMJ.* 2004; **329**: 1488–92.

21 Muir Gray JA. Evidence-based medicine for professionals. In: Edwards A, Elwyn G, editors. *Evidence-Based Patient Choice.* Oxford: Oxford University Press; 2001. pp. 19–33.

22 Abbasi K. Compulsory registration of all clinical trials. *BMJ.* 2004; **329**: 637–8.

23 Cook DJ, Mulrow CD, Haynes BR. Systematic reviews: synthesis of best evidence for clinical decisions. *Ann Intern Med.* 1997; **126**: 376–80.

24 www.nicsl.com.au/cochrane/guide_whatiscl.asp (accessed May 2008).

25 Davis DA, Thompson MA, Oxman AD *et al.* Changing physician performance: a systematic review of the effect of continuing medical education strategies. *JAMA.* 1995; **274**: 700–5.

CHAPTER 8

Personal development and self-care

This chapter explores:
- the importance of looking after oneself – healthy lifestyles
- doctors' morbidity and mortality
- the reasons why doctors get sick
- fear of failure versus the imposter syndrome
- burnout
- what doctors do when they are ill
- improving well-being
- health promotion and disease prevention
- the doctor's doctor
- diagnosis and recognition of problems.

> . . . Staff work best for patients when they can strike a healthy balance between work and other aspects of their life outside work.
>
> *Department of Health*[1]

> A doctor who treats him- or herself has a fool for a doctor and an idiot for a patient.
>
> *Sir William Osler (1849–1919)*[2]

Over 10 years ago Liam Donaldson, who later became Chief Medical Officer for the Department of Health, defined some of the issues that arise when doctors become ill[3] (*see* Box 8.1). 'Duty' and 'protecting patients' are integral to professionalism, and therefore issues relating to sickness in doctors and ways in which doctors should maintain their health are important topics to cover in our discussion. As with other sectors of society, certain conditions and diseases are deemed more acceptable than others, and more worthy of sympathy and compassion. A doctor who is stricken by multiple sclerosis is likely to be treated with respect compared with one who has a mental illness or an addiction such as alcoholism. Moreover, our patients react in some strange ways when they hear of their doctor's misfortune. Some find the information 'amusing', in that a doctor cannot heal himself, while others are more concerned that their own care will be compromised because their familiar physician is absent. GPs feel that patients do not want to consult a doctor who is sick, as the doctor's state of health reflects the doctor's competence.[4]

BOX 8.1 CONSIDERATIONS WHEN DEALING WITH SICK DOCTORS

- The need to protect patients.
- The duty of other doctors to report problems.
- The responsibility of the employer to care for its staff.
- The legitimacy given to some types of chronic illness and not others.
- The question of whether doctors should be regarded as special cases.

Doctors are expected to know what to do to prevent or minimise ill health. Yet many patients know of the saying that an alcoholic is someone who drinks more than his doctor. Part of the professional medical persona is to be healthy, while maintaining a lifestyle that includes dedication to the job (sometimes for 24 hours a day) and superhuman interpersonal skills.

MAINTAINING ONE'S HEALTH

Doctors and health professionals should practise what they preach! There is no need to list all the advice we give to patients about healthy lifestyles, but a quick summary reminds us of how we don't always follow our own suggestions. Don't smoke, drink alcohol in moderation only, take regular exercise, maintain a healthy weight, eat seven portions of fruit and vegetables every day, take time to relax and have regular holidays from work, spend time with the family, have regular screening for those conditions for which screening tests are available, and don't ignore signs of ill health. However, doctors are not superhuman, and we have all the excuses our patients do – too busy, don't enjoy exercise, running is not for me, the odd drink won't hurt (every day and double at weekends), alcohol helps me to relax, I can't stand my children so why would I want to spend time with them, I need more money, holidays are stressful, and so on.

Does the overweight doctor who wheezes up the steps to the surgery present a professional image to his or her patients? Is it professional behaviour to arrive five minutes late for every clinic because of a hangover from the night before? Is it just being approachable and down to earth to spend a few hours in the pub most nights where a lot of your patients hang out?

Doctors and health professionals also need to consider what they do when suffering from an acute self-limiting illness. Although many patients seem not to notice when their doctor is coughing and sneezing, perhaps this is also not the best professional image for a doctor to project. What would one tell a patient in this condition who was working in the public sector? But so many of us struggle on, first with minor illnesses and then with major ones. Our patients couldn't manage without us, could they?

SICK DOCTORS

The mortality and morbidity data relating to doctors are interesting. Male doctors overall have a significantly lower mortality rate than the general male population, but are more likely to die from suicide, liver cancer or cirrhosis.[5] Doctors are known to be at high risk of mental health problems compared with other professionals.[6] Depression, anxiety, substance abuse and alcoholism are relatively common among the profession, as well as post-traumatic stress disorder, panic disorder and obsessive-compulsive disorder.[7] The proportion of doctors and health professionals who suffer from above-threshold levels of stress is about 28% in most studies, compared with 18% of the general working population.[8] A report by the British Medical Association in 1998 stated that about 1 in 15 doctors during their lifetime might become dependent on drugs or alcohol.[9] Doctors who retire early from clinical practice are more likely to do so because of mental health rather than physical health problems.[10]

Stressed doctors are more likely to make mistakes. Some of this risk is compounded by lack of sleep, although tiredness in itself is not stressful if the doctor feels supported and valued.[8] Once a mistake has been made, the doctor is likely to feel more stressed, and so the vicious cycle continues. Moreover, the process of having a complaint made against oneself is a major stressor, even if it is eventually decided that the doctor did not in fact make an error. Some mistakes haunt doctors all their lives.[11]

The Department of Health, in the document *Taking Alcohol and Other Drugs out of the NHS Workplace*, states that 'drug or alcohol misuse by anyone working in the NHS is wholly unacceptable.'[12] This is due to the potential for harm to patients, staff and visitors. Drugs and alcohol impair performance and contribute to social, economic and domestic problems. Hospital and primary care trusts are responsible for setting up and monitoring a substance misuse policy, while staff are reminded that they have a duty of care for their colleagues. The Department of Health urges employees to self-refer if they believe that they have a problem. The recommendation to employers is not to invoke automatically disciplinary action for voluntary referral where the employee successfully undergoes a programme of treatment. However, concern has been expressed that this publication has led to addicted doctors being even more reluctant to seek help from their peers than they were previously.[7]

CAUSES OF ILL HEALTH

The Nuffield Trust has identified four main precipitating factors that account for doctors' poor health records,[13] to which others may be added from experience (*see* Box 8.2).

BOX 8.2 FACTORS THAT AFFECT DOCTORS' HEALTH

- The 'complex psychodynamics of doctor–patient relationships.'[14]
- Long hours of working.
- High workload.
- Pressures relating to work.
- Effects of these pressures on personal lives.
- Dealing with uncertainty.
- Perfectionism.
- Inability to switch off after work.
- Living with another health professional.
- Easy access to medication (including free samples and returned medication).
- Alcohol playing a major part in socialising with peers.
- Concerns that taking time off will affect career progression.
- Not wanting to let the team down by being absent.
- Discrimination.
- Coping with examinations.
- Examination failures.

Many of these factors are difficult to combat (e.g. examinations, the nature of the job with its attendant stresses). Some are being addressed through legislation (e.g. long working hours, high workload, discrimination), while others need to be addressed personally (e.g. alcohol consumption, self-medication). Long working hours are an interesting topic and the subject of some debate. Within the European Union the number of hours thought to be acceptable for doctors to work has been slashed by the European Working Time Directive to a maximum 48 hours in 7 days. In the USA, an 80-hour working week is considered to be fairly normal. In an editorial in *Medical Education*, the contrast in attitudes to such discrepancy in work patterns is amusingly told. A doctor who came back 'after hours' to deliver a baby is thought by American peers to be an example of the altruistic professional who puts his patients first, whereas Scandinavian medical educators, who are used to a 40-hour week, see such behaviour as unprofessional as it negates the principles of self-care and the balance between personal and working life.[15]

People who choose to become doctors are high achievers in general, and often find it hard to cope with failure, yet medical school and higher professional examinations can be difficult to pass. These assessments might be the first that these bright young people have ever failed in their lives. Even if they pass, their grade or class position may not be as high as they expected. 'Average' is not usually a word that has been used to describe them, and an adjustment is needed but is sometimes not made.

THE IMPOSTER SYNDROME

Conversely, many high achievers suffer from what has been called the 'imposter syndrome.' This phenomenon was first described by the psychologists Clance and Imes in 1978.[16] Taking a psychotherapeutic look at high-achieving women, they postulated that little girls are socialised from an early age into thinking that their achievements are the result of luck or sympathy, whereas boys' successes are due to talent or hard work. However, the imposter syndrome has since been recognised in both men and women.[17] There are two psychometric scales for its detection – the Clance Scale[16] and the Harvey Scale.[17]

As with any syndrome there is a collection of symptoms, including feelings of inadequacy that persist even when there is evidence to the contrary, such as high examination scores, promotion or the award of an honour. The affected person continues to have chronic self-doubt and a fear that all of their credentials will be rescinded once they are inevitably found to have been fraudulently obtained. From personal experience, many medical students and doctors appear to have varying degrees of the condition. It seems to recur when other stresses are high. One characteristic that appears to belong to the syndrome is a recurrent dream that some important examinations are to be held the next day and the candidate (the dreamer) has done no revision for them. This dream does not help to induce a peaceful night's sleep.

In one study of medical, dental, nursing and pharmacy students, 30% of respondents were found to have experienced imposter syndrome. Moreover, the imposter score was the strongest predictor of stress in medical students.[18] An American survey of family medicine residents found an even higher incidence among women doctors (41%) and a smaller incidence among male doctors (24%). The imposter syndrome symptoms were strongly correlated with anxiety and depression.[19]

The imposter syndrome seems to be a feature of professionalism that perhaps needs to be discussed and watched for in training programmes. Signs of the condition include students saying that their examination passes are 'down to luck', or doctors downplaying their achievements with what appears to be false modesty – 'It was nothing' or 'The examiner must have been having a good day.' The fear of being found out often means that the person cannot enjoy his or her success. Students and junior doctors need to be advised of the condition and challenged when they make self-deprecating remarks.

UNHAPPY OR BURNT OUT?

In 2001, Richard Smith, the previous editor of the *British Medical Journal*, asked 'Why are doctors so unhappy?'[20] He cited many reasons for the epidemic of miserable doctors, including overwork and lack of support, as well as adverse media coverage and high patient expectations. He also suggested that the government was likely to diagnose the doctors' malady as resulting from diminished control and increased accountability (i.e. aspects of de-professionalisation). However, his conclusion was that there is a 'mismatch between what doctors are trained for and what they are required to do . . . trained in pathophysiology, diagnosis and treatment, doctors find themselves spending more time thinking about issues like management, improvement, finance, law, ethics and communication.'[20] Again, some of these issues are directly related to professionalism.

Training in these areas may therefore improve doctors' mood and thus their performance. Another suggestion is that there should be more careful selection of medical students, as personality traits even at this early stage of career development predict those doctors who are more likely to become less satisfied, more unhappy, more stressed and ultimately burnt out.[21]

When does unhappiness become burnout? Burnout is mainly a problem of professional life, and doctors are at high risk. The condition consists of physical and/or emotional exhaustion due to prolonged stress or frustration. Symptoms are diverse and include many that are linked to anxiety and depression (*see* Box 8.3).

BOX 8.3 SYMPTOMS OF BURNOUT

- Feeling tired/tired all the time.
- Not wanting to go to work, or dreading going to work.
- A sense of doom.
- Poor communication with patients and peers.
- Resenting patients or feeling hostile towards them.
- Difficulty in caring for others.
- Working too quickly or too slowly.
- Feeling tearful.
- Feeling anger towards team members.
- Feeling put upon or the hardest worker in the team.
- Taking time off work.
- Feeling that what you do is useless.
- Feelings related to the 'imposter syndrome.'

DOCTORS' HEALTH-SEEKING BEHAVIOUR

It is not only the ill health itself of doctors that causes concern, but also what doctors do when they or their families become ill. The British Medical Association has produced guidelines for sick doctors, which may be regarded as the professional standard on what to do when a doctor or their relative needs medical help.[22] The guidelines are also the policy of the General Medical Council. The clear message is that doctors should not treat themselves or their families (*see* Box 8.4).

BOX 8.4 ETHICAL RESPONSIBILITIES OF
DOCTORS TOWARDS THEMSELVES[22]

- It is not advisable for doctors to assume responsibility for the diagnosis and management of their own health problems or those of their immediate family, except in the most unusual circumstances.
- All doctors should be registered with a general practitioner.
- As with all other patients, the responsibility for overall care and continuity

of treatment for doctors and their families should rest with their GP.
Referral for consultant advice or care should be made through their GP.

- It is not advisable for doctors, including professional suppliers, to prescribe themselves anything other than over-the-counter medicines.
- Doctors need to be aware that they become the patient in the doctor–patient relationship when they are receiving medical care.
- Doctors have an ethical duty to themselves and to their patients to ensure that their own health problems are effectively managed, to seek competent professional advice, particularly on their ability to work, and to follow this advice.

A survey conducted in 1999 by the Centre for Health Services Studies at the University of Kent looked at whether doctors were following these guidelines as patients. The majority of doctors who responded (96%) stated that they were registered with a GP. However, most of them never consulted their GP.[23]

Many doctors continue to work when physically, psychologically or spiritually unfit to do so. In the UK, an audit of junior doctors found that almost 75% were reluctant to take sick leave for infectious diseases because of concern about colleagues having to do extra work, while around 20% cited consultant pressure as a barrier to taking time off.[24] In some situations, when doctors are self-employed, sick leave may have a detrimental effect on income, causing even more stress. Thus as well as risking damaging their own health, sick doctors are potential sources of iatrogenic infection to patients.

The Australian Medical Association also recommends that every doctor should have a general practitioner.[25] Yet a survey of 358 Australian doctors in 2003 found that only 55% of respondents had their own GP, 71% were embarrassed to seek help from another doctor, 25% felt that it was acceptable to treat their own chronic conditions, and 95% were likely to work when sick.[26] Similar patterns and attitudes have been found among junior doctors in Australia.[27]

A study of GP registrars carried out by the Department of General Practice and Rural Medicine at James Cook University in Australia, involving 273 registrars over a period of 4 years, found that 11.4–18.1% of the registrars had health issues at some time in their training, but only 6.7%–9.8% saw a GP. The health issues included infectious illnesses, medical conditions, pregnancy and psychological problems.[28] A qualitative analysis of 33 registrars from the same cohort found that 32 doctors felt that their GP training had had a medium or strong negative effect on their psychological health, while a smaller number reported physical problems such as muscle tension and high blood pressure.

Only six of these doctors had sought help from their own GP, while 11 doctors had used self-help measures.[29]

Self-medication is common, particularly among those doctors who have ready access to analgesics, including opioids (e.g. anaesthetists, emergency physicians and psychiatrists).[30] In the Kent survey mentioned above, 71% of GPs and 76% of consultants admitted that they 'usually' or 'sometimes' self-prescribed. Self-prescribing of opiates, anxiolytics, antidepressants and hypnotics has been found to occur in 10% of GPs and 15% of consultants.[23] Junior doctors show similar behaviour. In an American survey of residents, 52% of respondents reported self-prescribing. A high proportion of the drugs that were self-prescribed (42%) came from a samples cupboard, and 11% came from pharmaceutical company representatives.[31] Thus there will be no records of much of the medication that doctors take. Overall, studies show that doctors are reluctant to seek healthcare through the usual mechanisms, and find it difficult to adopt the role of patient.[4]

The question arises as to when this behaviour starts. Is it during medical training? According to a study conducted by the Nuffield Provincial Hospitals Trust, attitudes that are formed at medical school are one of the reasons why doctors do not seek help later in their careers.[32] Each year papers are published documenting medical students' stress and its causes. Although medical students appear to experience more stress than non-students of similar ages,[33,34] they are not necessarily more stressed than other student groups.[35] Stress among medical students is precipitated by studying, and by worries about progress and aptitude.[36] It is associated with low levels of social support.[32]

Little is known about the physical health of students, or about their help-seeking behaviour in relation to both physical and mental health problems. Studies tend to look at the role of the medical school in monitoring and improving student welfare, mainly with regard to mental distress[37,38] and the importance of stress management programmes,[39] rather than the role of GPs in support and management of students suffering from physical and mental ill health. One North American study of 1027 students from nine medical schools across the USA found that 90% of respondents felt that they had needed healthcare during medical school. Nearly half of them reported difficulty obtaining healthcare due to being too busy to take time off (37%), concerns about cost (28%), concerns about confidentiality (15%), and having no access to healthcare (4%). Two-thirds of the students had obtained informal care from colleagues, and half of them had asked a colleague to perform a physical examination.[40] Medical students report barriers to seeking help with regard to their health, and are more likely to seek advice informally from friends and/or family with regard to mental healthcare.[41]

Informal care from colleagues is part of the culture of the medical profession, and perhaps it is something that students pick up from their clinical role models. It is known that medical students do learn attitudes and values from their clinician role models, and that these role models are a powerful force in the learning process.[42]

In the UK, with its strong system of general practice, it would be hoped that medical students would access help for physical and mental health problems from a GP. However, there are other issues to consider. Once a person becomes a medical student, the attitudes of other health professionals towards that person change. A medical student is no longer a layperson. Little is known about this transition from layperson to doctor and the way that it affects help-seeking behaviour.

INITIATIVES TO IMPROVE WELL-BEING

The Department of Health's *Improving Working Lives Standard* is a blueprint for NHS employers and staff, demonstrating commitment to improving the working life of all employees, including health professionals. Since March 2006, all NHS organisations have been required to show that they are implementing the standard. Some of the elements to be made available are listed in Box 8.5. An online questionnaire survey of UK hospital doctors in 2005 found that more support is still needed to improve their working lives. Senior doctors want better secretarial and managerial support, while junior doctors have requested improved education, training and mentoring. Female doctors require improved childcare facilities.[43]

BOX 8.5 IMPROVING WORKING LIFE

- Greater flexibility and control over own time.
- Flexible careers.
- Flexible retirement.
- Training and development.
- Improved access to childcare.
- Encouragement of diversity.
- Tackling discrimination, harassment and bullying.
- Team working.
- Healthy working.
- Improved communication.

Strategies to improve working life should also help to reduce the incidence of burnout and mental health problems. Other interventions include mentoring and appraisal.[21] The way in which appraisal is promoted and carried out within the workplace is important, as the process itself can be stressful. Effective appraisal by skilled individuals should identify those doctors or other health professionals who are unhappy, demotivated, stressed or heading towards burnout.[44] However, there also need to be processes in place to help such individuals once they have been identified.

The way in which medical error is handled is also important in order to reduce the risk of long-term damage to a professional's mental health. Whether the mistake comes to light through observation by a colleague or following a complaint by a patient, the process needs to be handled with sensitivity and empathy. The complaints procedure is often unwieldy and a long, drawn-out affair, during which time a doctor can lose confidence. The ability to handle some incidents at a local practice level in the case of GPs is important for speeding up the inquiry. However, one of the Shipman Inquiry recommendations was that all complaints should be made known to the local primary care organisation (PCO).[45] Although this may help to reveal a pattern of poor performance, it is also likely to increase stress and reduce well-being in many doctors.

EDUCATION AND PREVENTION

Practising doctors do not feel that self-care was taught adequately at either undergraduate or postgraduate levels.[4] These days, medical schools in their personal and professional development courses usually include some teaching about self-care (*see* Chapter 10). It is important that issues such as abuse of alcohol and prescribed and illegal drugs are discussed. Many medical students overindulge in alcohol. Pub crawls, cheap drinks nights and drinking games are all part of the social life of university – and this in the context of a rise in binge drinking among *all* young people in the UK. Faculty staff look on these behaviours fairly favourably in general, whereas other recreational drug use is not condoned at all. However, heavy drinking patterns established early on in medical students' careers may cause trouble in later life. Moreover, non-alcohol-drinking students are often marginalised by this culture, and this may cause poor team working.

Students also need to be encouraged to talk about mental health issues. They should know where to seek confidential help, as many of them will be unfamiliar with the place where they are studying. They may not know how to register with a doctor away from home.

Many of us remember suffering from hypochondriasis when we were at medical school. Medical students who are learning about symptoms and diseases often believe that they have all kinds of conditions, both common and exotic. Most of the time they ignore their worries and learn to live with their shifting diagnoses. However, some do seek help, and the doctor's attitude to them is important in establishing how they perceive health-seeking behaviour in the future. Spiro and Mandell from Yale University School of Medicine feel that this hypochondriasis has other long-term effects, as it 'contributes to easy denial, because then physicians fear one disease after another and find them all phantom, they come to believe in their own invulnerability. Only unrelenting pain, great weight loss, catastrophic bleeding . . . awaken them to the reality that they have become patients.'[46]

Talking things over is one way of helping to relieve the stresses caused by clinical practice. Many doctors use 'black' or 'gallows' humour to reduce the often overwhelming emotions that they experience when confronted by human suffering, the inability to make a difference, death and dying. However, support and recognition of these emotions are also necessary. Junior doctors do not often talk to senior staff about their reactions to the death of a patient, yet they are often powerfully affected by such common occurrences.[47] This lack of discussion may lead to poor coping mechanisms, overtime burnout and mental health problems.[48]

LEARNING FROM DOCTORS', HEALTH PROFESSIONALS' AND ONE'S OWN STORIES

> The stories of sick doctors force emotion back into medicine, and when sick doctors themselves learn the comfort that comes from attention and devotion, empathy cannot lag far behind.[46]

The Personal View column in the *British Medical Journal* often consists of accounts of doctors' illnesses and what was learned from the experience. Although the doctor usually gains an insight into what it means to be sick, frequently there is also a subtext of how things might have been handled differently.

Many doctors do learn empathy from their own misfortune, particularly if they are able to reflect on the experience. Learning may also occur by proxy. Thus narratives of illness are useful learning tools for facilitating discussion by students and doctors of what it means to be ill and how patients might be feeling in similar situations. Empathy – that is, the ability to be affected by something which happens to another person, not oneself – may be learned. A distinction may be made between natural empathy and empirical empathy.[49] The former does not require a personal experience of suffering, but rather the ability to imagine what another person is going through, while the latter is the positive outcome of distressing or painful experiences. Doctors' tales of illness recount their narrators' acquisition of empirical empathy.

Most doctors and health professionals have personal experiences that may promote empirical empathy. Students and junior doctors are less likely to have had such experiences, and therefore there is a trend within medical and other health professions education to integrate the humanities into the curriculum. Students may learn from novels, non-fiction and other media how patients react to illness, bereavement and other life events.

ACTING AS A DOCTOR'S DOCTOR

Dealing with sick colleagues and hearing their stories at first hand it seems that, as with most things in medicine, there is no one right way of interacting with fellow professionals. Some want to adopt a sick role completely, have responsibility taken away, and be treated as if their medical knowledge was no greater than that of the average person. In particular, doctors from one specialty need to remind other specialists that they require explanation of terms and treatments just as much as any other patient. Information sharing at the right level is important. Other doctors like to retain their professional personas and downplay their conditions – they view being ill as somehow weak, and will not admit to pain or anxiety.

Sick doctors may act out the patients whom they perceive as 'perfect.' Think of your favourite patients – they don't complain, they submit to procedures without moaning, they put up with pain and rarely request extra analgesia, they don't ask awkward questions or challenge authority, they apologise for calling their doctor at night, they say 'please' and 'thank you', and they show their gratitude with gifts. Being a doctor's doctor is difficult. Both doctor-patient and doctor-doctor are watching each other. Both are anxious in case they slip up. The shared decision making that is difficult with non-professional patients is even more so with colleagues. Asking for the doctor-patient's opinion may be seen as being uncertain or wanting authority: 'A judicious paternalism may be in order.'[46]

If a colleague *does* ask for medical advice, this should be offered in a formal setting and not in a corridor consultation or at a social gathering. Box 8.6 suggests ways of conducting a consultation with a colleague. The British Medical Association recommends that 'it is preferable that a doctor's

GP should not be a relative, nor, if at all feasible, a partner of the doctor.'[22] This is difficult in some locations where there may only be one practice. The University of Kent survey found that around 25% of the GPs were registered with a partner in their practice. There is obviously conflict between the two roles of working partner and GP, as advising the patient to take time off will increase the workload of the partner.[23]

BOX 8.6 CONSULTATIONS WITH COLLEAGUES[50]

- Discuss confidentiality and clarify the physician–patient relationship as early as possible.
- Perform thorough examinations in formal circumstances.
- Ask about self-treatment and self-diagnosis and discourage these practices.
- Discuss diagnostic and treatment plans in detail. Do not assume that a physician's professional knowledge makes such discussion unnecessary.
- Avoid engaging in corridor consultations, but do not refuse to help a colleague who is ill. Instead, encourage the colleague to seek appropriate help.

RECOGNISING PROBLEMS IN ONESELF AND OTHERS

Self-care involves prevention of ill health by taking measures to adopt a healthy lifestyle and reduce stress by healthy means (i.e. not through the use of drugs and alcohol). However, it also involves recognising that when one is ill, one's performance is impaired and patients are at risk. Then something needs to be done!

It is hard to make an appointment to see a GP and to discuss one's health. Physical symptoms are perhaps easier to talk about, but doctors worry about appearing to be hypochondriacs. Communicating about stress is difficult, as any doctor will realise that his or her physician is likely to be facing similar work pressures. However, the underlying professional duty is to seek help, treatment and/or sick leave before any patient receives substandard care or is harmed.

Perhaps a colleague needs to suggest that you ought to see a doctor. Any such suggestion should be taken seriously. Conversely, if you are worried about a colleague, that concern should be acted upon. What happens next partly depends on the problem. It should be fairly easy to approach a colleague who seems to have a physical illness, whereas it is more difficult if the signs are pointing to alcohol or drug abuse. Of course you never know if your colleague is already receiving help. However, the GMC guidelines are clear – if a doctor thinks that patient care is being compromised by the actions or health of another doctor, it is not sufficient to adopt a 'wait and see' policy[51] (*see also* Chapter 9).

SUMMARY

Professionalism involves a doctor or health professional taking care of their own health, partially to act as a role model for patients, but also in order to fulfil their professional role at the highest standard. The nature of clinical work is such that health professionals are at high risk of experiencing stress and mental health problems. There are various measures that can be adopted both personally and institutionally to reduce these risks. Every doctor should have a GP and seek medical help when necessary. Doctors who are looking after their colleagues need to be professional about this and should insist that their 'doctor as patient' consults within a proper appointment.

SOURCES OF HELP

BMA Counselling Service (for BMA members only). Tel: 08459 200169.
National Counselling Service for Sick Doctors (NCSSD). Tel: 020 7306 3272.
Doctors' Support Network; www.dsn.org.uk

REFERENCES

1 Department of Health. *Improving Working Lives Standard*; www.dh.gov.uk/en/Managingyourorganisation/Humanresourcesandtraining/Modelemployer/Improvingworkinglives/index.htm (accessed May 2008).
2 Bennett Bean W, editor. *Sir William Osler: aphorisms from his bedside teaching and writings*; www.vh.org/adult/provider/history/osler/1.html (accessed May 2008).
3 Donaldson LJ. Sick doctors. *BMJ.* 1994; **309:** 557–8.
4 Thompson WT, Cupples ME, Sibbett CH *et al.* Challenge of culture, conscience and contract to general practitioners' care of their own health: qualitative study. *BMJ.* 2001; **323:** 728–31.
5 Office of Population Censuses and Surveys. *Occupational Health Decennial Supplement.* London: HMSO; 1995.
6 Williams S, Michie S, Pattani S. *Improving the Health of the NHS Workforce. Report of the partnership on the health of the NHS workforce.* London: Nuffield Trust; 1998.
7 Stanton J, Caan W. How many doctors are sick? *BMJ Career Focus.* 2003; **326:** S97a.
8 Firth-Cozens J. Doctors, their wellbeing and their stress. *BMJ.* 2003; **326:** 670–71.
9 British Medical Association. *The Misuse of Alcohol and Other Drugs by Doctors: a report*

of the working group on the misuse of alcohol and other drugs. London: British Medical Association; 1998.

10 Pattani A, Constantinovici N, Williams S. Who retires early from the NHS because of ill health and what does it cost? A national cross-sectional study. *BMJ.* 2001; **322:** 208–9.

11 Mizrahi T. Managing medical mistakes: ideology, insularity, and accountability among internists in training. *Soc Sci Med.* 1984; **19:** 135–46.

12 Department of Health. *Taking Alcohol and Other Drugs out of the NHS Workplace.* London: Department of Health; 2001.

13 Nuffield Trust. *Taking Care of Doctors' Health: reducing avoidable stress and improving services for doctors who fall ill.* London: Nuffield Provincial Hospital Trust; 1996.

14 Chambers R, Maxwell R. Helping sick doctors. *BMJ.* 1996; **312:** 722–3.

15 Hodges BD, Segouin C. Medical education: it's time for a transatlantic dialogue. *Med Educ.* 2008; **42:** 2–3.

16 Clance PR, Imes SA. The imposter phenomenon in high-achieving women. *Psychother Treat Res Pract.* 1982; **15:** 241–7.

17 Harvey J, Katz C. *If I'm So Successful, Why Do I Feel Like a Fake? The imposter phenomenon.* New York: St Martin's Press; 1985.

18 Henning K, Ey S, Shaw D. Perfectionism, the imposter phenomenon and psychological adjustment in medical, dental, nursing and pharmacy students. *Med Educ.* 1998; **23:** 456–64.

19 Oriel K, Plane MB, Mundt M. Family medicine residents and the imposter phenomenon. *Fam Med.* 2004; **36:** 248–52.

20 Smith R. Why are doctors so unhappy? *BMJ.* 2001; **322:** 1073–4.

21 Peile E, Carter Y. Selecting and supporting contented doctors. *BMJ.* 2005; **330:** 269–70.

22 British Medical Association. *Ethical Responsibilities Involved in Treating Doctor-Patients.* London: British Medical Association; 1995.

23 Forsythe M, Calnan M, Wall B. Doctors as patients: postal survey examining consultants' and general practitioners' adherence to guidelines. *BMJ.* 1999; **319:** 605–8.

24 Perkin MJ, Higton A, Witcomb M. Do junior doctors take sick leave? *Occup Environ Med.* 2003; **60:** 699–700.

25 NSW Doctors' Mental Health Implementation Committee. *Doctors' Mental Health Policy.* Sydney: NSW Health Department and NSW Branch, Australian Medical Association; 1997.

26 Davidson SK, Schattner PL. Doctors' health-seeking behaviour: a questionnaire survey. *Med J Aust.* 2003; **179:** 302–5.

27 Shadbolt N. Attitudes to healthcare and self-care among junior medical officers: a preliminary report. *Med J Aust.* 2002; **177:** S19–20.

28 Larkins SL, Spillman M, Vanlint J *et al. Stress, Personal and Educational Problems in Vocational Training: a prospective interventional cohort study. Final report.* Townsville, Queensland: James Cook University; 2002.

29 Larkins SL, Spillman M, Parison J *et al. Flexibility, Isolation and Change in Vocational Training for General Practice. A qualitative analysis of personal and educational problems experienced by a subgroup of general practice registrars.* Townsville, Queensland: James Cook University; 2002.

30 Bennet J, O'Donovan D. Substance misuse by doctors, nurses and other healthcare workers. *Curr Opin Psychiatry.* 2001; **14**: 195–9.

31 Christie J, Rosen I, Bellini L *et al.* Prescription drug use and self-prescription among resident physicians. *JAMA.* 1998; **280**: 1253–5.

32 Nuffield Provincial Hospitals Trust. *The Provision of Medical Services to Sick Doctors: a conspiracy of friendliness?* London: Nuffield Provincial Hospitals Trust; 1994.

33 Stecker T. Well-being in an academic environment. *Med Educ.* 2004; **38**: 465–78.

34 Adams J. Straining to describe and tackle stress in medical students. *Med Educ.* 2004; **38**: 463–4.

35 Singh G, Hankins M, Weinman JA. Does medical school cause health anxiety and worry in medical students? *Med Educ.* 2004; **38**: 479–81.

36 Moffatt KJ, McConnachie A, Ross S *et al.* First-year medical student stress and coping in a problem-based learning medical curriculum. *Med Educ.* 2004; **38**: 482–91.

37 Tennant CC. A student mental health and welfare program in a medical school. *Med J Aust.* 2002; **177**: S9–10.

38 Dahlenburg GW. Conference overview: a duty of care. *Med J Aust.* 2002; **177**: S3–4.

39 Shapiro S, Shapiro D, Schwartz G. Stress management in medical education: a review of the literature. *Acad Med.* 2000; **75**: 748–59.

40 Roberts LW, Warner TD, Carter D *et al.* Caring for medical students as patients. *Acad Med.* 2000; **75**: 272–7.

41 Brimstone R, Thistlethwaite JE, Quirk F. Health help-seeking behaviour of medical students. *Med Educ.* 2007; **41**: 74–83.

42 Wright S. Examining what residents look for in their role models. *Acad Med.* 1996; **71**: 290–2.

43 Dornhorst A, Cripps J, Goodyear H *et al.* Improving hospital doctors' working lives: online questionnaire survey of all grades. *Postgrad Med J.* 2005; **81**: 49–54.

44 Conlon M. Appraisal: the catalyst of personal development. *BMJ.* 2003; **327**: 89–91.

45 Smith J. *Fifth Report. Safeguarding Patients: lessons from the past – proposals for the future.* London: The Shipman Inquiry; 2004.

46 Spiro HM, Mandell HN. When doctors get sick. *Ann Intern Med,* 1998; **128**: 152–4.

47 Redinbaugh EM, Sullivan AM, Block SD *et al.* Doctors' emotional reaction to recent death of a patient: cross-sectional study of hospital doctors. *BMJ.* 2003; **327**: 185.

48 Association of Professors of Medicine. The well-being of doctors. *Am J Med.* 2003; **114**: 513–19.

49 Mathiasen H, Alpert JS. Lessons in empathy: literature, art and medicine. In: Spiro H, Curnan MGM, Peschel E *et al.*, editors. *Empathy and the Practice of Medicine.* New Haven, CT: Yale University Press; 1993.

50 www.webmm.ahrq.gov (website of the USA-based Agency for Healthcare Research and Quality) (accessed May 2008).

51 General Medical Council. *Duties of a Doctor: good medical practice.* London: General Medical Council; 1995.

CHAPTER 9

The nature of autonomy for the professional and the patient

This chapter explores:
- professional autonomy
- self-regulation, autonomy and the GMC
- changes to the GMC
- the continuing saga of revalidation
- whistleblowing
- complaints against doctors
- the introduction of clinical audit and clinical governance
- factors that contribute to potential de-professionalisation
- the patient as consumer.

The central element of professional autonomy is the assurance that individual physicians have the freedom to exercise their professional judgement in the care and treatment of their patients. . . . The World Medical Association and its National Medical Associations re-affirm the importance of professional autonomy as an essential component of high-quality medical care and therefore a benefit due to the patient that must be preserved . . . as a corollary to the right of professional autonomy, the medical profession has a continuing responsibility to be self-regulating. In addition to any other source of regulation that may be applied to individual physicians, the medical profession itself must be responsible for regulating the professional conduct and activities of individual physicians.

The World Medical Association, 1987[1]

One of the defining characteristics of a profession is its autonomy – the condition of self-government and, deriving from this, its right to self-regulation. In recent years, for a number of reasons, the medical profession has been under threat with regard to its autonomy. However, the nature of this autonomy is complex, and is not simply a question of who has the power to chastise a doctor, remove a doctor's right to practise or inflict conditions on a doctor's method of working. Certainly in the UK the relationship between state and medical profession is intimately connected to the way in which the profession operates within its sphere of influence. British doctors have never been wholly free from state control, as was shown within the historical context in Chapter 2. The nature of the state–profession relationship and its bearing on autonomy will be explored further in this chapter.

Changes in professional power and regulation have been occurring in tandem with developments in the way in which patients interact with healthcare providers. The concepts of patient autonomy, patient partnership, patient safety, consumerism, citizenship and patients' charters all have effects on the way in which medicine is practised. The question is what is the nature of the impact of such patient empowerment on the autonomy of the medical profession? Audit, clinical governance and increasing accountability are affecting professional behaviour. What are the benefits, if any, for patients in this brave new world of transparency and data gathering?

PROFESSIONAL AUTONOMY

Professional autonomy, in theory, relates to all six elements of a profession (*see* Chapter 1). However, we have to ask to what extent the medical profession may truly claim to be autonomous while being subject to state control. Freidson suggested that doctors are entirely subordinate to the state in terms of the social and economic constraints of their work, but have sole control over the technical aspects.[2] Moreover, such autonomy and monopoly are only possible because of their dependence on and sponsorship by the state.[3] This analysis has been challenged on the basis that state and profession are more intimately connected than Freidson surmised. The French psychologist and philosopher Michel Foucault (1926–1984), whose prolific works include analyses of the interaction between society and medicine, believed that the professions and the modern state developed together, the former being a product of the latter's policies.[4] According to Foucault, 'governmentality' (his word for the process of governing that evolved in Europe) encompasses all of the technical expertise, knowledge, mechanisms and institutions that exist within a state. The modern professions are the institutionalised form of that expertise. Thus the professions emerged concurrently with the modern state, and the state gave them official recognition as experts.

This conclusion, according to Professor Johnson, sociologist at Leicester University, means that when we try to understand what is happening between the state and the professions we should not think solely in terms of tension between professional autonomy and state intervention. As Johnson points out, because of this symbiotic relationship between professionalisation and state formation, 'any modern government that pursues policies with the effect of politicising established areas of expertise and destabilising existing professional jurisdictions also risks undermining the entrenched conditions that sustain legitimate official action.'[5] Put simply, if there is too much state interference in medical matters, public trust of doctors will be lost and the government's medical agenda will be undermined. If patients feel that doctors are trying to meet government targets because of political pressure rather than altruism, the nature of the doctor–patient relationship built on trust will be adversely affected. It is thus advantageous to the government to allow the profession a degree of professional autonomy – not only in clinical matters but also in regulation of behaviour and training. It also means that the profession, or any other strong and organised group, 'may continue to stand between the individual and state and when necessary oppose it.'[6]

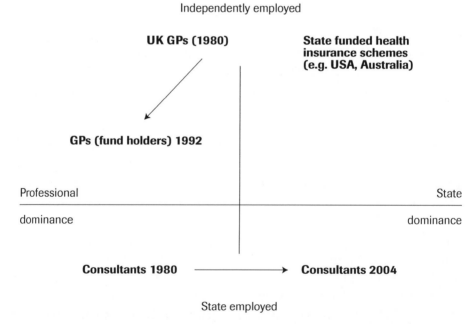

FIGURE 9.1 Changing relations of doctors with the state (adapted from Light[7]).

Donald Light, Professor of Comparative Healthcare Systems in New Jersey, views this interaction between state and profession as one of countervailing powers. The two bodies go through phases of harmony and discord during which countervailing actions take place in a time frame of years to decades.[7] During this time, professional dominance and state dominance wax and wane. Light has produced a model to illustrate this process, which highlights how the position of even subsets of doctors (GPs, specialists) varies with the political climate (*see* Figure 9.1).

According to this model, general practitioners in the UK gained some dominance at the expense of independence when the Conservative Government introduced fundholding in 1992. The GP contract of 2004 probably moved them back towards their 1980 position, although the introduction of practice-based commissioning (PBC), if successfully implemented, will leave those who take up this process somewhere between the two points. (A survey in 2007 showed that 54% of general practices had agreed a commissioning plan with their primary care trust[8]). The UK consultants moved to the right on the graph because of the 'primary care-led NHS', and subsequently a new contract that emphasised the importance of audit, performance review and detailed description of job plans.

Most of these changes were first unveiled in *The NHS Plan: a plan for investment, a plan for reform*, published by the Department of Health in 2000. This document outlined the new contracts for both general practitioners and hospital consultants, which came into force a few years later. The plan aimed to introduce 'a new system of earned autonomy' which 'will devolve power from the Government to the local health services as modernisation [of the NHS] takes hold.'[9]

THE GENERAL MEDICAL COUNCIL AND SELF-REGULATION

Meg Stacey, a sociologist at Warwick University, wrote a history of the GMC in 1992. Her research explored how the GMC attempted to balance maintaining unity within the profession, which she feels is essential for any self-regulatory function, and protecting the public.[10] Her evidence suggests that the professional agenda came first. This was corroborated by Sir Donald Irvine (president of the Council between 1995 and 2002) in his book *The Doctors' Tale*, a personal account of turbulent times at the GMC. The book documents the emergence of a new ethos of professionalism and the challenges to professional regulation.[11]

As we saw in Chapter 2, the GMC was founded in 1858 and currently works under the aegis of the 1983 Medical Act. Although it is a statutory body, it is independent of the state. The Council is financed by the fees paid by doctors who register annually in order to practise within the UK. It controls this register of doctors and also decides what qualifications are needed for such registration. Approval of medical school curricula and method of examination is also the GMC's responsibility. Up until 2004, annual retention on the GMC's list was simply a matter of a doctor paying the fee following full registration, after obtaining a university degree and working as a pre-registration house officer (or intern) for one year. A doctor could be removed from the register only for failing to pay the money or if he or she was found guilty of gross professional misconduct or was deemed unfit to practise. Doctors could be referred to the GMC for disciplinary action by various bodies, including other doctors, patients and following legal proceedings in court. The GMC thus did not react until things went wrong. There was also a culture of secrecy about doctors' personal conduct and their clinical performance. In a 2003 lecture (later expanded in his book), Sir Donald Irvine concluded that 'this was a profession used to seeing patients' interests through its own eyes and on its own terms.'[12]

BOX 9.1 CHANGES AFFECTING SELF-REGULATION INTRODUCED AFTER THE BRISTOL INQUIRY

- Introduction of mandatory clinical audit.
- Clinical standards defined.
- Revalidation to ensure clinical competence is maintained.
- Framework for assessing professional performance.
- Definition of responsibility within team-based care.
- Research into complex systems and how they succeed or fail.
- Better system of informed consent.
- Measures to improve communication skills of doctors, particularly in relation to discussion of risk.
- Importance of patient safety emphasised, and measures to ensure this.
- Emphasising the importance of doctors monitoring their colleagues' clinical activity and taking prompt action once problems are diagnosed.

Challenges to the power of the GMC followed two major medical scandals in the 1990s. The Bristol case centred on paediatric cardiac surgery and the deaths of 30 children under the age of 1 year, many of which were probably preventable, over a period of a decade. The report on the tragedy, which was published in 2001 following a public inquiry,[13] precipitated widespread changes in the way that the GMC functions. Irvine spoke of the Bristol Inquiry as giving 'insights into the darker side of the profession's culture.'[11] The public exposure of the attitudes of the profession to audit, team working, consent to treatment and complaints against poor practice led to a major loss of public confidence in doctors' ability to regulate their practice. Richard Smith, editor of the *British Medical Journal* until 2004, saw the fallout of the case as being a decrease in trust between individual patients and doctors, as well as between society and doctors' organisations.[14] Dr Smith used Yeats' words, 'All changed, changed utterly', for the title of this seminal editorial. The repercussions of the Bristol case and inquiry directly affect professionalism. Many of the measures introduced in the last decade are a direct result of the Bristol Inquiry. Some of them would have happened anyway, but the Government's response was quick and far-reaching (*see* Box 9.1).

The other recent major case to challenge the profession in the UK was the conviction of the Hyde GP Harold Shipman in 2000, initially for murdering 15 of his patients with intravenous opiates. It is now believed that he killed over 300 patients over a 24-year period. The Shipman Inquiry, conducted by Dame Janet Smith, generated six reports. The conclusion with regard to the GMC was that historically it had acted more to support doctors than to protect the interests of patients. The fifth report called for increased monitoring of the work of GPs, including prescribing, particularly of controlled drugs, and greater control over death certification.[15] The GMC responded by publishing the document *Developing Medical Regulation*,[16] which outlined a four-layer model for self-regulation in the future, summarised by Graeme Catto, President of the GMC (*see* Box 9.2).[17]

BOX 9.2 THE FOUR LAYERS OF REGULATION

- *Personal regulation:* or self-regulation by individuals who are committed to a code of ethical conduct and put patients first.
- *Team-based regulation:* which requires health professionals to take responsibility for the teams in which they work, and means that they should report a team member's poor performance or health problems.
- *Workplace regulation:* the responsibility of healthcare providers to ensure the fitness to practise of their staff.
- *Professional regulation:* by the GMC and other health professional bodies, including education, registration and revalidation.

THE ROLE OF PUBLIC INQUIRIES

Walshe and Higgins from the Manchester Centre for Healthcare Management have written a comprehensive review of the use and impact of inquiries within the NHS.[18] They cite the five major inquiries of the last few years: the Bristol Inquiry and the Harold Shipman Inquiry already discussed above, plus an inquiry into security at Ashworth Hospital Secure Unit near Manchester, the case of the gynaecologist Rodney Ledward, and the scandal of retention of babies' body parts at Alder Hey Hospital. The purposes of such public inquiries are to establish the facts of these high-profile cases, to reassure the public that any breach of professional conduct will be strictly dealt with, to demonstrate the accountability of the profession and to learn lessons from the failings that are uncovered. However, as Walshe and Higgins point out, these inquiries often have similar findings (*see* Box 9.3), demonstrating that lessons are not learned and systems failures are not always remediated.

BOX 9.3 COMMON FINDINGS IN PUBLIC INQUIRIES[18]

- Inadequate leadership.
- Organisational or geographical isolation that hinders peer review.
- System or process failures.
- Lack of or poor communication both between team members and between doctors and patients.
- Disempowerment of staff and patients; discouragement of raising of concerns.

Although medical errors are often caused by a series of systems errors rather than by individual mistakes,[19] major changes in the regulation of doctors arising from these cases aim to improve both system and individual practitioner problems.

The National Patient Safety Agency was established in 2001 as a 'special health authority' within the NHS, with the overall purpose of co-ordinating efforts to report and, more importantly, to learn from and prevent mistakes that affect patient safety.[20] The National Clinical Assessment Authority (NCAA), which was also set up in 2001, is a body designed to help hospitals and trusts that have concerns about the performance and professional behaviour of individual doctors.[21] Finally, the Commission for Health Improvement (CHI), also set up in 2001 and now called the Commission for Healthcare Audit and Inspection, has a remit to investigate serious instances of failure within the health service.[22]

THE GMC UP TO 2008

In 1951, Parsons suggested that 'the physician is a technically competent person whose competence and specific judgements and measures cannot be competently judged by the layman.'[23] However, total self-regulation is no longer feasible, and the membership of the GMC now includes 14 lay members elected by the Privy Council. They join 19 doctors elected by their peers who are registered with the GMC, and two academics representing the Royal Colleges and the universities. This 'new-look' GMC was reconstituted in 2003.

David Jewell, editor of the *British Journal of General Practice*, has summed up the problem facing the GMC after Shipman: 'Operating in the public domain, and with direct accountability to Parliament as well as intermittent formal review of its procedures . . . it can only damage itself and the profession if it allows any actions to be interpreted as acting leniently to underperforming doctors.'[24]

In 2004, the GMC began to introduce a system of revalidation. The proposal was that doctors would have to show that they remain competent to practise, including being involved in continuing professional development/education, and that their knowledge and skills are up to date. (Continuing professional development is discussed in more detail in Chapter 7.)

REVALIDATION

The GMC's initial plans for revalidation were overturned by concerns raised by the fifth report of the Shipman Inquiry.[15] Dame Janet Smith has stipulated that the GMC must identify poorly performing doctors as well as certifying that a doctor has the right positive attributes. The current system of annual appraisal of doctors in the UK, which was introduced in 2003, was not intended to detect substandard medical care, and was always viewed as a formative and developmental process. However, it could be used together with clinical governance as 'reliable mechanisms for delivering a positive demonstration of individual doctors' fitness to practise.'[25] Professor Mike Pringle has suggested in the 2005 John Fry Fellowship Lecture various ways of collecting evidence about fitness to practise that together will constitute revalidation. As well as appraisal, these include the results of case-based and conventional audits, an annual reflective personal development plan, 360-degree assessment by patients and peers, certification of clinical skills such as communication and cardiopulmonary resuscitation, and self-certification of health.[26] Some of these issues will be picked up and developed further in Chapter 11, which looks at assessment of professionalism.

The document *Good Doctors, Safer Patients*[27] by the Chief Medical Officer of Health (published in July 2006) acted as a consultation document to be accepted in whole or in part as a blueprint for revalidation by the GMC. The emphasis was on the protection of patients through a regulatory process that is feasible and non-punitive. The recommendation is for two levels of revalidation – relicensure, so that a doctor may remain on the medical register, and recertification, so that a doctor may remain on the relevant specialist register. Relicensing will be based on a new system of appraisal. Recertification will be a function of the Royal Colleges, which will need to define standards and identify assessment tools. Specialist certification will need to be renewed every five years.

Paragraph 44 of the final chapter is worth quoting in full:

> It is important to ensure that the concept of medical regulation is not limited to the identification of poor practice. Arguably, debate and effort have concentrated on designing a system to deliver this objective, and thus the discussion on the future of medical regulation has been more negative and confrontational than it needed to be. Although one of the prime purposes of medical regulation must be to protect the safety of patients, it must also be the true guardian of professionalism. The regulatory system must be able to demonstrate that all practising doctors reach specified standards, which may themselves evolve over time to reflect changes in patterns of work, technology and the expectations of society.[27]

THE GMC IN THE TWENTY-FIRST CENTURY

In February 2007, the Department of Health produced a White Paper building on *Good Doctors, Safer Patients* that finally set out the reforms under which the GMC will lose the right to regulate the medical profession. *Trust, Assurance and Safety: the regulation of health professionals in the 21st century*[28] envisages a yet smaller GMC with equal numbers of lay and medical members. Although it will continue to set standards for professional conduct and investigate doctors who have been accused of serious misconduct, it will no longer decide whether doctors who are found guilty of such misconduct will be allowed to continue to practise. This responsibility will pass to a separate, independent tribunal with legal, lay and medical members. Judgements on fitness to practise will also be made on the basis of the civil standard of probabilities rather than on the criminal standard of 'beyond reasonable doubt', as was the case before.

The GMC will still continue to accredit education for undergraduates and continuing professional development. (Post-qualification training becomes the responsibility of the Postgraduate Medical Education and Training Board.) Revalidation will occur every five years.

WHISTLEBLOWING: WHAT DO YOU DO AND HOW DO YOU DO IT?

The *Oxford English Dictionary* defines whistleblowing as 'to bring an illicit activity to an end by informing on [the person responsible].'[29] This is an interesting concept for two reasons. First, within the NHS most whistleblowing involves raising concerns about a process or system rather than about an individual. Secondly, in the past many whistleblowers have been treated unfairly and suspended or sacked without the activity stopping (see, for example, an article by Revill published in *The Observer* in 2003[30]). Both the Government with its 'Public Disclosure Act',[31] which protects whistleblowers, and the GMC[32] have acted to give confidence to concerned employees. All NHS organisations should now have a whistleblowers' policy with transparent lines of responsibility to a senior management level. Critical incident forms are useful for outlining what facts and evidence are needed. The GMC regards whistleblowing as a *professional responsibility*: 'You must protect patients when you believe that a doctor's or other colleague's health, conduct or performance is a threat to them.'[33] However, because of the risk to physical and psychological health from speaking up for standards,[34] it is advisable to seek legal or defence body advice before taking action. Many professionals will probably be cautious about taking any action if they remember the case of Steve Bolsin, the whistleblower at Bristol. Bolsin, a junior consultant anaesthetist, was ostracised and virtually driven out of the UK following disclosure of his well-founded concerns, and is now practising in Australia.[35]

Coull, writing in *Careers BMJ*, has listed several gambits that organisations use to stall whistleblowers[36] (*see* Box 9.4). His article is amusing but has a hard edge.

BOX 9.4 ORGANISATIONAL STRATEGIES THAT ARE USED AGAINST WHISTLEBLOWERS (ADAPTED FROM COULL[36])

- Discrediting the messenger.
- Stalling until the person moves jobs.
- Making the whistleblower feel foolish by saying that no one has ever raised such an issue before.
- Transference of blame by suggesting that patients will suffer if an inquiry is held.

- Saying that something will be done and then ignoring the issue and hoping that it will go away.
- Being patronising and insinuating that the whistleblower cannot possibly understand the wider picture.
- Threatening the whistleblower with loss of job, reference and/or career.

COMPLAINTS AGAINST DOCTORS BY PATIENTS

Patients make complaints about doctors for several reasons. Often they simply want to know exactly what went wrong and why. Lack of communication and miscommunication are thus common precipitating factors in complaints. Sometimes they want an apology and/or reassurance that their problem will not occur again, either to themselves or to others. And of course they might want financial recompense.

Complaints should be made within a year of the problem arising or of the patient being aware of a problem. The best outcome certainly for the doctors is local resolution at the hospital trust or general practice level. Each general practice must have a complaints system. If the patient is not satisfied with this process, a lay conciliator may be appointed to discuss the case with the patient and the doctor concerned. Thereafter if resolution is not achieved, the patient has 28 days in which to request an independent review. Here again lay people are involved in the matter – a lay chair approved by the Secretary of State works with two clinical assessors, a convenor and a local representative of the organisation involved. The next stage is to involve the ombudsman, who will make recommendations for change based on the findings of their investigation.

Patients may, of course, refer a doctor directly to the GMC. The GMC acts in cases of 'serious professional misconduct' (conduct which makes the GMC question whether the doctor should be allowed to continue to practise medicine without restriction), when a doctor has been convicted of a criminal offence, when a doctor fails on several occasions to meet required professional standards, and when a doctor has an illness or condition that affects his or her ability to practise (e.g. mental illness, alcohol or drug abuse). The GMC will issue a warning, but as outlined above can no longer strike a doctor off the medical register. This power is being passed to an independent tribunal. The GMC cannot award compensation. The patient must take the doctor to court if they wish to sue. The GMC publishes guides for patients[37] and doctors[38] about the referral process.

The NHS Litigation Authority, established in 1995, is responsible for handling negligence claims against NHS bodies. Such a complaint takes on average 1.44 years to resolve, causing stress to all involved. Between 2006 and 2007 there were 5426 claims of clinical negligence and 3293 claims of non-clinical negligence, a small decrease compared with the previous year.[39] However, despite popular belief and the myth of a 'compensation culture', and although the number of complaints is rising, the number of negligence claims is not increasing.[39]

CLINICAL AUTONOMY AND CLINICAL AUDIT

Tolliday has identified four components of clinical autonomy[40] (*see* Box 9.5). Clinical autonomy may also be viewed as the freedom of the medical profession to define the needs of patients and to use state/health service resources to meet those needs[41] – technical expertise in Freidson's analysis. In the early days of the NHS, these privileges were safeguarded by doctors who did not accept any accountability for the way that such resources were used. A doctor's decision about a management plan was sacrosanct. Other doctors might discuss the best way to treat X or Y, but the decision was based on clinical grounds rather than on cost-effectiveness. Moreover, the clinical grounds were not necessarily evidence based, but related to a doctor's past experiences, favourite drugs, adverse reactions in previously managed patients and, cynically, inducements from pharmaceutical companies and advertising. Until the mid-1980s, GPs did not think about the cost of their referrals to the secondary sector. As the gatekeepers of the NHS, they played an important role in deciding who should receive specialist care, but the decision as to whom and where to refer was a GP's alone, regardless of expense. In fact most doctors would have no idea how much an individual referral cost the state, nor whether there were any differences in price between specialists in various parts of the country.

BOX 9.5 FOUR ELEMENTS OF CLINICAL AUTONOMY[40]

- The right to independent practice.
- The right to refuse to treat an individual patient.
- The responsibility to lead and co-ordinate other health professionals.
- The overarching primacy of medical knowledge.

The Conservative Government challenged this state of affairs, initially in the 1980s, when it recognised that 80% of overall health costs were generated by the medical decisions of doctors.[42] Although clinical audit had been suggested as early as the 1960s, and had been the subject of a Royal Commission and subsequent report in 1979,[43] the medical profession had been reluctant to undertake such activity for the state. The Conservatives' White Paper of 1989, *Working for Patients*, ensured that audit was introduced.[44] The 'new GP contract'[45] of 1990 included a requirement that GPs must provide practice activity data and produce annual reports. This increased surveillance meant that the state had greater control over the work of GPs.[46] There were financial incentives to provide business plans and improve practice management. Since then clinical audit, and more recently clinical governance, have been a feature of life within the NHS. The Labour Government set up the National Institute for Clinical Excellence (NICE) in 1999 to make recommendations to the NHS in England and Wales on new technologies and new drugs, to produce or approve clinical guidelines, and to encourage quality improvement.[47] The NICE definition of clinical audit is shown in Box 9.6. Audit is about improving the quality of service and clinical delivery to patients, but of course there is an underlying aim to reduce costs and improve efficiency. Indeed Richard Smith, previous editor of the *British Medical Journal*, criticised NICE itself as being primarily about rationing healthcare.[48]

BOX 9.6 A DEFINITION OF CLINICAL AUDIT[49]

Clinical audit is a quality improvement process that seeks to improve patient care and outcomes through systematic review of care against explicit criteria and the implementation of change. Aspects of the structure, processes and outcomes of care are selected and systematically evaluated against explicit criteria. Where indicated, changes are implemented at an individual, team or service level, and further monitoring is used to confirm improvements in healthcare delivery.

All consultants and GPs are now under contract to undergo regular audit of their practice as a condition of service. This accountability has been seen as a threat to clinical autonomy. A medical audit model derived from the systems model of Donabedian is shown in Figure 9.2.

Clinical governance (*see* Box 9.7) was conceived in the 1997 document *The New NHS*.[51] Since then all health organisations have had a statutory duty to seek quality improvement through clinical governance. The hallmark of a well-managed organisation is defined as the integration at every level of clinical quality, financial control and service performance. Defining clinical quality is more difficult and open to debate. Obviously such clinical quality should be a requirement of a professional's daily work. The World Health Organization lists four elements of quality (*see* Box 9.8), including patients' perspectives on the care provided. High quality of care means that health services for both individuals and populations increase the likelihood of the desired health outcomes, which are consistent with current professional knowledge – that is, interventions that work applied to the right patient at the right time.[52] For a doctor to have current professional knowledge, to be 'up to date' with medical research and evidence, a system of continuing professional development is necessary (*see* Chapter 7).

Structure	Process	Outcomes
System characteristics (e.g. hospitals, general practices)	Technical style	Clinical end points (e.g. morbidity, mortality)
Provider characteristics (e.g. doctors, allied health professionals, qualifications of staff)	Interpersonal style, including communications skills	Patients' satisfaction with care
Patient characteristics (e.g. acute, chronic, age)		Functional status, quality of life
		General well-being

FIGURE 9.2 Donabedian's model of medical audit.[50]

BOX 9.7 A DEFINITION OF CLINICAL GOVERNANCE[51]

Clinical governance is a system through which NHS organisations are accountable for continuously improving the quality of their services and safeguarding high standards of care by creating an environment in which excellence in clinical care will flourish.

BOX 9.8 WORLD HEALTH ORGANIZATION DEFINITION OF CLINICAL QUALITY[53]

- Technical quality: professional performance.
- Efficiency relating to the use of resources.
- Risk management (the risk of injury or illness associated with the service provided).
- Patients' satisfaction with the service provided.

DE-PROFESSIONALISATION?

De-professionalisation, which is an ugly word for an interesting concept, may be viewed as 'a reduction in occupational privileges.'[54] The previous analysis of how the state and the medical profession are intimately connected in the UK suggests that de-professionalisation to any great extent is unlikely. Light's theory of countervailing forces views what is happening to the medical profession not as de-professionalisation, but as a reaction by the state (the profession's partner) to the dominance of the profession leading to excesses and imbalance.[7] These imbalances are listed in Box 9.9.

BOX 9.9 IMBALANCES PRECIPITATING THE STATE'S INTERVENTION[7]

- Internal elaboration and expansion that weaken the profession from within.
- Subsequent tendency to consume more and more of a nation's wealth.
- Self-regarding importance that ignores patients' concerns (and those of the partner-government).
- The degree and nature of competition with allied professions (e.g. nurses, complementary practitioners).
- The changing technological base of its expertise.
- The demographic composition of its membership.

Within this climate it is easy to think of examples of state interference in the technical or clinical aspects of medical practice (*see* Box 9.10). Although most of these have been decided in consultation with practising doctors, the impetus for the control came from the government. It is unlikely that GPs and specialists would have suggested all such measures themselves. However, it is also true that GPs have been given increasing clinical freedom in other areas in which traditionally they have been restricted compared with their hospital colleagues. For example, GPs now have open access to investigations such as most X-rays, gastroscopies and hysteroscopies for which patients previously had to see a specialist for ratification of the request prior to the investigation being carried out. Some of this freedom dates from fundholding and the power of the GP to set contracts and conditions of practice with the hospitals. Fundholding GPs certainly had more clinical autonomy than their non-fundholding colleagues, a circumstance that caused professional divisions at the time.

BOX 9.10 RESTRICTIONS ON CLINICAL AUTONOMY IN THE UK

- The 'black list' (drugs that cannot be prescribed, introduced under NHS regulations in 1985).
- Prescribing of certain new drugs being limited to hospital specialists.
- Some drugs being restricted to patients with defined conditions (e.g. Viagra).
- Limits to the number of particular drugs that may be prescribed in a certain time.
- No open access by GPs for certain new investigative procedures.
- IVF restricted to women of a certain age and parity.

However, in the last decade, in parallel with the decrease in professional autonomy there has also been a decrease in respect for doctors by individual patients and the general public. At a very simplistic level we see this in the case of home visits. In 'the old days' GPs tell us patients would put out a clean towel and a new bar of soap for the doctor. Nowadays, GPs are lucky if the television is switched off. However, although most patients think well of their own personal doctor, 'this level of respect and trust does not extend to the profession's institutions, where the public perception is of self-interest arising from a failure to make self-regulation work for all patients.'[12]

BOX 9.11 POSSIBLE REASONS FOR THE PUBLIC'S LOSS OF FAITH IN DOCTORS

- Financial inducements for immunisations and smears – 'clinical targets.'
- Removal of patients from GPs' lists because of 'refusal' by patients to have their children immunised.
- Reluctance of GPs to make home visits.
- Deputising services for out-of-hours medical care.
- From 2005, an end to the 24-hour commitment by GPs, and difficulty obtaining medical help outside office hours.
- Surgery hours not being 'user-friendly' for working people.
- Changes in the way that patients are able to make appointments.
- Lengthening waiting lists.
- Apparent decline in doctors' altruistic calling.

A number of disparate factors may be cited as the reasons for the medical profession's fall from its position of respect, and the critical reaction of people to what has been perceived as doctors' arrogance (*see* Box 9.11). Doctors have been vilified in the media, often with just cause, but also with little concrete evidence of any wrongdoing. The big medical stories such as those of Bristol, Alder Hey and Harold Shipman are well known. There has also been a steady publication of lesser events, but whose numbers have a cumulative effect on public opinion. Stories of doctors' 'mistakes' are commonplace – failure to diagnose, wrong prescriptions, sex scandals and refusal to see patients make the headlines. Popular magazines include 'readers' stories' of medical mishaps, in which the doctor's side of the story is rarely heard. Doctors are also seen by some as greedy. They make a lot of money compared with many patients, but they still seem to want more for doing less.

The GP contract of 2004 included financial incentives for what many would think of as routine aspects of a doctor's work, such as measuring and reducing patients' blood pressure, giving advice about smoking cessation, and secondary prevention of ischaemic heart disease by the prescription of aspirin. These are examples of what Freidson calls 'conflicting methods' of organising a healthcare system.[55] The government assumes that doctors can be motivated to change their practice by 'purely self-interested, material incentives.' However, there is an underlying assumption that, as professionals, doctors will act for the well-being of their patients and base their decisions on doing good, rather than on monetary reward. This tension may also be seen in the discussion between parent and doctor about childhood immunisation. The parent may well ask 'Is my GP persuading me to consent to this immunisation for the well-being of my child or because she wants to meet her target and receive more pay?' Such erosion of trust threatens the mystique of professionalism and the traditional doctor–patient relationship.

PATIENT AUTONOMY AND THE RISE OF CONSUMERISM

The NHS Plan envisaged a health service designed around the patient.[9] Patients are in general now better informed than they were up to the later years of the twentieth century. Patients – who regularly access the Internet, read about medical discoveries in the newspapers, and watch popular science programmes on television – want a greater say in their management. The doctor's opinion is often only one of many that a patient has explored. Many doctors find it hard to cope with challenges to their 'professional' judgements, and feel that the patient empowerment movement has gone too far. One result of this is the rising number of complaints against doctors, many due to lack of communication. In the past doctors did not need to explain. They ordered patients to 'take the tablets', and usually the patients did (and if they didn't, the patients rarely admitted this). With a rise in the number of private fee-paying patients in the UK, the balance of power has also shifted. Private patients tend to get longer appointments and expect more dialogue with the person whose services they are buying.

The Patient's Charter of 1991 defined the rights of patients and the standards of service that they should expect within the NHS.[56] This charter-led health service led some doctors to fear that efficiency and giving in to patients' unreasonable demands would be more important than providing services to sick people.[57] Health professionals now express concern about the rise of 'consumerism' in medicine. Some equate 'patient choice' and 'patient partnership' with a free market in which patients may demand their rights regardless of evidence, cost or suitability. However, within a national health or insurance-funded service, patients will never be consumers in the accepted sense of the word (i.e. a person who purchases goods and services for personal use[25]). Freidson[55] has suggested that there are three ways in which the market of health services may be organised (*see* Box 9.12). Non-fee-paying patient choice is limited by what is available through the health service or, in the USA, by what the insurance companies are prepared to finance. Under such circumstances, healthcare cannot be offered through a free market in which patients are true consumers. Nor is the bureaucratic model ideal, as it relies on uniformity and standardisation, whereas patients need to be treated as individuals whose outcomes are often unpredictable. The professional model is the ideal for health services.

BOX 9.12 HEALTH SERVICES MARKET MODELS[55]

Free market
- Workers compete freely to be employed.
- Workers are paid by employers or clients.
- Consumer is in command.
- Common interest is price (lowest for consumer).
- Employers' and workers' interest is gain/profit.
- Aim is to reduce cost of labour and production in order to increase profits.

Bureaucratic market (e.g. state-owned utilities)
- Organised and controlled by a hierarchy.
- Manager or executive is in command.
- Aim is to have reliable and predictable production of specified goods or services.

- Price is less important than reliability.
- Quality is defined by formal standards.
- Performance of workers is evaluated.
- Consumer can only choose between what the bureaucratic officials have decided to produce.
- Workers compete for jobs and advancement.
- Pay is less important than career, job security and working conditions.

Professional market

- Organised and controlled by the professionals themselves.
- Professional member is in command.
- Workers need licences to work, controlled by profession.
- Emphasis is on their community and collegiality.
- There are set incomes which are protected.
- Commitment to do work well and to gain approval from fellow professionals.
- Value of work is not evaluated by cost but by quality.
- 'Consumer' is limited to those allowed to work.

MAINTAINING PROFESSIONALISM

In this analysis, Freidson describes professionalism as follows: 'Competition is focused around the virtuosity and quality of work that gains the honour and respect of colleagues and symbolic rewards such as awards and citations, in which financial gain is a marginal consideration.'[55] However, compared with the free market, this model does not mean that patients cannot and should not be involved in decisions about healthcare. They may be involved at an individual level, through the process of shared decision making in which doctors discuss the available options, and at a local and/or national level, by being involved in the planning of services to decide availability. The professional market is built on trust – trust between members and the trust of the patient in the professional performance of the doctor, including their competence, behaviour and attitude.

This is why professionalism is worth preserving, but the criticism shows that it needs to be rethought and to evolve. Doctors' entrenched attitudes to status and paternalism, where they are still present, must be challenged. The conduct of the medical profession must be open to evaluation and regular inspection. We must be accountable to informed public opinion and admit our mistakes.

SUMMARY

Professionalism involves autonomy and self-regulation. These processes are no longer wholly tenable in today's health service. However, the movement towards greater accountability, clinical governance and lay involvement in complaints procedures should not be thought of as 'de-professionalisation.' Patients are becoming partners in their healthcare, and this extends to expecting professional conduct, so when this is lacking, patients should be included in any regulation or investigation of complaints. Doctors must be accountable both to their peers and to their patients, working within the state system and answerable to the state and the population.

REFERENCES

1 World Medical Association; www.wma.net/e/policy/a21.htm (accessed May 2008).
2 Freidson E. *Profession of Medicine: a study in the sociology of applied knowledge.* New York: Dodd, Mead and Co.; 1970.
3 Larson MS. *The Rise of Professionalism: a sociological analysis.* Berkeley, CA: University of California Press; 1977.
4 Foucault. M. Governmentality. In: Burchell G, Gordon C, Miller P, editors. *The Foucault Effect: studies in governmentality.* Hemel Hempstead: Harvester Wheatsheaf; 1991.
5 Johnson T. Governmentality and the institutionalisation of expertise. In: Johnson T, Larkin G, Saks M, editors. *Health Professions and the State in Europe.* London: Routledge; 1995. pp. 7–24.
6 Stacey M. The British General Medical Council. In: Johnson T, Larkin G, Saks M, editors. *Health Professions and the State in Europe.* London: Routledge; 1995. pp. 116–38.
7 Light D. Countervailing powers. A framework for professions in transition. In: Johnson T, Larkin G, Saks M, editors. *Health Professions and the State in Europe.* London: Routledge; 1995. pp. 25–41.
8 www.dh.gov.uk/en/Publicationsandstatistics/Statistics/DH_082156 (accessed February 2008).
9 Department of Health. *The NHS Plan: a plan for investment, a plan for reform.* London: The Stationery Office; 2000.
10 Stacey M. *Regulating British Medicine: the General Medical Council.* Chichester: John Wiley & Sons; 1992.
11 Irvine D. *The Doctors' Tale: professionalism and public trust.* Oxford: Radcliffe Medical Press; 2003.
12 Irvine D. *Patient-centred professionalism – decision time* (Duncan Memorial Lecture, 2003); www.mja.com.au/public/issues/181_05_060904/inv10434_fm.pdf (accessed May 2008).
13 Public Inquiry into Children's Heart Surgery at the Bristol Royal Infirmary, 1984–1995. In: *Learning from Bristol.* London: The Stationery Office; 2001.
14 Smith R. All changed, changed utterly. *BMJ.* 1998; **316:** 1917–18.

15 Smith J. *Fifth Report. Safeguarding Patients: lessons from the past – proposals for the future.* London: The Shipman Inquiry; 2004.

16 General Medical Council. *Developing Medical Regulation: a vision for the future.* London: General Medical Council; 2005.

17 Catto G. Professionalism pompous, pretentious and outmoded? *J Interprof Care.* 2005; **19**: 313–14.

18 Walshe K, Higgins J. The use and impact of inquiries within the NHS. *BMJ.* 2002; **25**: 895–900.

19 Reason J. Human error: models and management. *BMJ.* 2000; **320**: 768–70.

20 www.npsa.nhs.uk (accessed October 2005).

21 Department of Health. *Supporting Doctors, Protecting Patients.* London: Department of Health; 1999.

22 Department of Health. *A First Class Service: quality in the new NHS.* London: Department of Health; 1998.

23 Parsons T. *The Social System.* London: Routledge & Kegan Paul; 1951.

24 Jewell D. After Shipman: reforming the GMC – again. *Br J Gen Pract.* 2005; **55**: 83–4.

25 Lewis M. Mechanisms of revalidation. *Br J Gen Pract.* 2005; **55**: 640–41.

26 Pringle M. *Revalidation of doctors: the credibility challenge* (John Fry Fellowship Lecture). London: The Nuffield Trust; 2005.

27 Chief Medical Officer for Health. *Good Doctors, Safer Patients.* London: Department of Health; 2006.

28 Department of Health. *Trust, Assurance and Safety: the regulation of health professionals in the 21st century.* London: Department of Health; 2007.

29 Soanes C, Stevenson A, editors. *Oxford Dictionary of English.* 2nd ed. Oxford: Oxford University Press; 2003.

30 Revill J. Whistleblower lifts lid on NHS culture of secrecy. *The Observer*, 26 January 2003; www.guardian.co.uk/politics/2003/jan/26/nhs.health (accessed May 2008).

31 Office of Public Sector Information. *Public Interest Disclosure Act 1998.* London: The Stationery Office; 1998.

32 General Medical Council. *Maintaining Good Medical Practice.* London: General Medical Council; 1998.

33 General Medical Council. *Duties of a Doctor: good medical practice.* London: General Medical Council; 1995.

34 Lennane KJ. 'Whistleblowing': a health issue. *BMJ.* 1993; **307**: 667–70.

35 http://news.bbc.co.uk/1/hi/health/1384854.stm (accessed May 2008).

36 Coull R. Everything you always wanted to know about whistleblowing but were afraid to ask. *BMJ Career Focus.* 2004; **328**: S5–6.

37 General Medical Council. *Referring a Doctor to the GMC. A guide for patients.* London: General Medical Council; 2004.

38 General Medical Council. *A Guide for Doctors Referred to the GMC.* London: General Medical Council; 2004.

39 www.nhsla.com (accessed February 2008).

40 Tolliday H. Clinical autonomy. In: Jacques E, editor. *Health Services.* London: Heinemann; 1978.

41 Alaszewski A. Restructuring health and welfare professions in the United Kingdom.

In: Johnson T, Larkin G, Saks M, editors. *Health Professions and the State in Europe.* London: Routledge; 1995. pp. 55–74.

42 Dent M. Doctors, peer review and quality assurance. In: Johnson T, Larkin G, Saks M, editors. *Health Professions and the State in Europe.* London: Routledge; 1995. pp. 86–102.

43 Perrin J. *Management of Financial Resources in the National Health Service.* Royal Commission on the National Health Service. Research Paper No. 2. London: HMSO; 1978.

44 Department of Health. *Working for Patients.* London: HMSO; 1989.

45 Department of Health. *General Practice in the NHS: a 1990 contract.* London: HMSO; 1989.

46 Allsop J. The professional powers of GPs. In: Johnson T, Larkin G, Saks M, editors. *Health Professions and the State in Europe.* London: Routledge; 1995. pp. 75–85.

47 Rawlins M. In pursuit of quality: the National Institute for Clinical Excellence. *Lancet.* 1999; **353:** 1079–82.

48 Smith R. The failings of NICE. *BMJ.* 2000; **321:** 1363–4.

49 National Institute for Clinical Excellence. *Principles for Best Practice in Medical Audit.* Oxford: Radcliffe Medical Press; 2002.

50 Donabedian A. Evaluating the quality of medical care. *Milbank Memorial Fund Q.* 1996; **44 (Part 2):** 166–206.

51 Secretary of State for Health. *The New NHS.* London: The Stationery Office; 1997.

52 Scally G, Donaldson LG. Clinical governance and the drive for quality improvement in the new NHS in England. *BMJ.* 1998; **317:** 61–5.

53 World Health Organization. *The Principles of Quality Assurance.* Copenhagen: World Health Organization; 1983.

54 Larkin G. State control and the health professions in the United Kingdom. In: Johnson T, Larkin G, Saks M, editors. *Health Professions and the State in Europe.* London: Routledge; 1995. pp. 45–54.

55 Freidson E. *Professionalism Reborn: theory, prophecy and policy.* Cambridge: Polity Press; 1994.

56 Department of Health. *The Patient's Charter.* London: HMSO; 1991.

57 Herd B, Herd A, Mathers N. The wizard and the gatekeeper: of castles and contracts. *BMJ.* 1995; **310:** 1042–4.

CHAPTER 10

Learning and teaching professionalism

This chapter explores:
- key aims, principles and frameworks for education about professionalism
- outcome-based approach
- the hidden curriculum
- learning environment
- teaching communication, ethics and the law
- fostering self-awareness
- the role of humanities, creative writing and narrative approaches
- inter-professional learning approaches
- involving patients
- patient safety
- personal development plans, revalidation and appraisal
- the learner's perspective.

> The amount of clinical material required – in-patient and out-patient alike – depends obviously in part on the size of the staff, in part on the number of students; on reflection, it will be clear that it depends also on the method and theory of instruction.
>
> *Abraham Flexner, 1925*[1]

These days health professional educators who wish to enhance students' professional development would hopefully not refer to patients as 'clinical material.' Role models are so important in the context of learning and teaching professionalism that such terminology is a negative influence on professional attitudes.

CONTEXT

Historically, society assumed that most of the 'correct' professional attributes required of doctors (such as altruism, integrity, humanity and self-awareness) were already in place in the kind of people who were selected for medical school, and that they would pick up the rest from their teachers by a process of 'osmosis.' Indeed this often happened through the powerful process of role modelling, and the medium of the so-called 'hidden curriculum' (see below). However, student selection has, in the past, been based largely on academic achievement in science subject areas, which although predictive of *academic* achievement does not necessarily guarantee development of appropriate attitudes.[2] Furthermore, role modelling is by no means always a positive process, and the 'osmotic' transfer of attitudes and values can be unpredictable and inconsistent in its outcomes. Indeed it may even have detrimental effects, reinforcing negative and maladaptive behaviours and fostering cynicism. Thus, until relatively recently, medical students could graduate and qualify as doctors with very little formal education about professionalism. Although there might have been isolated courses on medical ethics, law and communication skills, there were few opportunities to reflect upon the underpinning values (including instances in which there might be value conflicts), or to think about what, as doctors, they should *be* (as opposed to what they should know or be able to do). Moreover, doctors could continue to practise medicine until retirement, and so long as they did not fall foul of the law for a serious offence – for example, get caught having sex with a patient, or taking prescription drugs not intended for them – they could more or less 'get away with murder' in terms of substandard care.

As we have seen, professionalism has been 'revisited' in the last decade or so, with changes in societal attitudes and developments in policy and practice driving educational change, as opposed to the converse (as is often the case). Thus educators have started to debate and discuss ways in which professionalism might be taught and learned. Indeed there has been a plethora of publications, working groups and consensus conferences addressing the subject. The bottom line is that few disagree that there *should* be formal and continuing education about professionalism. The debate centres around ways and means and, of course, how such learning might be assessed (*see* Chapter 11).

Stephenson and colleagues from King's College London defined some key aims for professional development during undergraduate training (*see* Box 10.1).[3] These aims are also adaptable and relevant for postgraduate training and continuing professional development (CPD).

BOX 10.1 KEY AIMS OF PROFESSIONAL DEVELOPMENT DURING MEDICAL SCHOOL[3]

- To enable students to understand the origins of professionalism and the proper set of responsibilities of the profession.
- To instil and nurture in students the development of personal qualities, values, attitudes and behaviours that are fundamental to the practice of medicine and healthcare.
- To ensure that students understand the importance and relevance of these concepts, demonstrate these qualities at a basic level in their work, and are willing to continue to develop their professional identity.

BOX 10.2 ESSENTIAL COMPONENTS OF EDUCATION ABOUT PROFESSIONALISM

Principles
- To be a professional is a privilege, not a right.
- Professionalism is an ideal to be pursued, with inherent moral value.
- Proper professional behaviour is essential for the healer to function and maintain trust.

Proposed content
Identifiable 'professionalism' content, including:
- clear definition of professionalism and its characteristics
- the separate but linked concepts of the 'healer' and the 'professional'
- codes of ethics, including their philosophical and historical derivations
- relevant material drawn from sociology, philosophy, economics and political science
- obligations to society that must be fulfilled in order to maintain public trust
- the nature of and relationship between individual and collective autonomy, and their limitations.

Learning process
- Introduced in undergraduate training, reinforced in postgraduate training.
- Part of assessment of all students.

Adapted from Cruess S, Cruess R. Professionalism must be taught. *BMJ*. 1997; **315**: 1674–5.[4]

Sylvia and Richard Cruess of Montreal have suggested that teaching about professionalism should include several components,[4] which can be summarised under the three headings of underlying principles, proposed content and learning process (*see* Box 10.2).

In the UK, the General Medical Council's guidance to medical schools on change in undergraduate curricula, *Tomorrow's Doctors*, was published in the early 1990s and was hugely influential in promoting change with regard to teaching and learning about professionalism. Explicit recommendations were made about ensuring that communication, ethics and medical law, and other relevant topics became part of the 'core' curriculum, that attention was given to inculcation of 'attitudes of mind and of behaviour that befit a doctor' and the personal and professional development of students, and that all of this, where possible, should be rigorously assessed.[5] A follow-up document, published in 2003, reiterated this guidance[6] and linked with another seminal GMC policy document, *Good Medical Practice*[7] (see below). It stated that 'The principles of professional practice set out in *Good Medical Practice* must form the basis of medical education', before going on to describe a set of learning outcomes based on these principles.[6] Similar educational developments have taken place across the globe – for example, in North America.[8]

Medical schools have responded over the past decade by developing and consolidating teaching and assessment in relevant areas, often drawing themes together into a coherent curricular strand. Such strands have names like 'Personal and Professional Development (PPD)', 'Values in Medicine' and 'Doctoring', and are now almost invariably part of the core curriculum. Although there is variation in content, the key elements of these courses usually consist of ethics and communication, team working and relevant material drawn from other disciplines, in line with the recommendations of Sylvia and Richard Cruess,[4] and aspects of 'how to look after yourself', including reflective practice. More recently, topics such as cultural diversity, patient safety and clinical governance have been incorporated into such strands.

At postgraduate level, a number of documents published by the General Medical Council, largely based upon *Good Medical Practice*, which was revised and updated in 2006,[9] provide a framework for continuing personal and professional development (*see* Box 10.3). *Good Medical Practice*, for example, is being used as the basis for appraisal, and for the curriculum for the Foundation Programme for newly qualified doctors in the UK.[10] It has been argued that these principles should not be seen as aspirational – achieved only by the best – but should be what *all* doctors attain.

BOX 10.3 PRINCIPLES AND ISSUES COVERED IN *GOOD MEDICAL PRACTICE* [9]

Good clinical care
- Providing good clinical care
- Supporting self-care
- Avoiding treating those close to you
- Raising concerns about patient safety
- Decisions about access to medical care
- Treatment in emergencies

Maintaining good medical practice
- Keeping up to date
- Maintaining your performance

Teaching and training, appraising and assessing
- Making assessments and providing references
- Teaching and training

Relationships with patients
- The doctor–patient partnership
- Good communication
- Children and young people
- Relatives, carers and partners
- Being open and honest with patients if things go wrong
- Maintaining trust in the profession
- Consent
- Confidentiality
- Ending professional relationships with patients

Working with colleagues
- Working in teams
- Conduct and performance of colleagues
- Respect for colleagues
- Arranging cover
- Taking up and ending appointments
- Sharing information with colleagues
- Delegation and referral

Probity
- Being honest and trustworthy

- Providing and publishing information about your services
- Writing reports and CVs, giving evidence and signing documents
- Research
- Financial and commercial dealings
- Conflicts of interest

Health
- If your health may put patients at risk

In Canada, the Royal College of Physicians and Surgeons published a similar framework, known as the 'CanMEDS Roles' (derived from 'Canadian Medical Education Directives for Specialists'), which lists core competencies for all doctors under the headings 'medical expert', 'communicator', 'manager', 'health advocate', 'collaborator', 'scholar' and 'professional.'[11] These now form the basis of accreditation, revalidation and CPD in Canada.

SOME EDUCATIONAL CONSIDERATIONS

Learning and teaching about professionalism, whether at undergraduate or postgraduate level, should conform to the following educational principles in order to maximise its relevance and effectiveness:[12]

➤ *'Learning in context'* motivates learners through its relevance, and can be achieved by ensuring that teaching about professionalism is grounded in the 'real world' – for example, relating it to real cases, taught and reinforced by clinical teachers.

➤ Teaching should be based as much as possible on *learners' experience* to bring issues to life, and to tap into a potentially rich vein of 'material.' In the context of professionalism this may be easier with more mature learners.

➤ *Promote reflection*, because experience alone can be a poor teacher if the learner does not have opportunities to reflect, especially in relation to attitudinal issues, value conflicts and development of self-awareness.

➤ *Integrate with other core learning and teaching* – again to promote relevance, but also so that concepts and principles are less easily marginalised by learners. Problem-first or case-led approaches obviously lend themselves to this.

➤ Teaching and learning should, where possible, be *evidence based* (in terms of both content and process). The evidence base of some subject areas that come under the heading of 'professionalism' is well established – for example, communication. For others, such as the value of inter-professional learning, the evidence base is less robust (see below).

➤ *Use a 'spiral' approach*, recognising that a 'once only' educational intervention is unlikely to have a lasting impact. Thus content should ideally be revisited and reinforced, at different levels and in different contexts.
➤ Finally, the teaching should be *practically oriented*, and focused on 'real-life' problems, again promoting relevance but also, in the postgraduate and CPD context, helping to address real learning needs.

In 2002, a workshop at an international conference in Lisbon generated a list of issues to guide development of professionalism, reiterating some of the above principles and proposing additional ones.[13] These include building a positive view of the importance of such training with all concerned (not least to promote a climate for change), using examples of good practice from other disciplines, matching teaching methods with intended learning outcomes, creating a learning environment that enables open, critical analysis of attitudes and behaviour to promote self-awareness, encouraging collaborative learning, formally assessing the learning (easier said than done; *see* Chapter 11), providing support and rewarding good performance in both learners *and* teachers, where possible incorporating the patient's voice, and finally ensuring that learners are exposed to positive role models.

Jill Gordon, Associate Professor of Medical Humanities at Sydney University, articulated and challenged some common objections to the introduction of professionalism into curricula.[14] These include the problem of curriculum overload, the view that the subject is not teachable, the view that specialist expertise is required to teach it, and the view that 'some things may be better left unsaid.'

A FRAMEWORK FOR DEVELOPING PERSONAL AND PROFESSIONAL DEVELOPMENT

Jill Gordon also proposed a framework to guide personal and professional development, based on the work of John Eisenberg, late Director of the United States Agency for Healthcare Research and Quality, and champion of evidence-based medicine and patient safety. This, she argued, could enable a more strategic and coherent approach to organising and delivering a professionalism curriculum, and thus avoid a piecemeal and fragmented approach.[14] The framework, shown in Box 10.4, plots factors that are known to influence behaviour against educational processes, including cognitive, affective and 'metacognitive' (i.e. reflective) processes. She suggests that this could help curriculum/course planners to identify gaps in their provision.

BOX 10.4 A FRAMEWORK FOR EDUCATION FOR PROFESSION

Factors influencing behaviour	Processes in learning		
	Cognitive	*Affective*	*Metacognitive*
Education	Provide a clear outline of professional requirements and standards; ethical and legal principles; ethical reasoning	Use personal experiences of patients, families and colleagues; provide evidence of benefits of PPD for patients, profession and healthcare system; harm done by lapses	Provide opportunities for reflection within formal teaching sessions, and adequate time for reflection outside formal teaching sessions
Feedback	Provide formative assessments of knowledge and reasoning	Give feedback on positive personal and professional behaviours from faculty, and encourage feedback from patients and colleagues	Give feedback that enables and encourages reflection, based on knowledge and understanding of students' needs
Rewards and incentives	Ensure cognitive mastery; include relevant PPD in other parts of the programme, especially clinical teaching; ensure that summative assessments reward knowledge	Remember the intrinsic rewards in satisfying altruistic drives and drives for self-actualisation; give extrinsic rewards, including encouragement by admired role models	Ensure that teaching rewards reflection (e.g. thoughtful discussion); create assessments such as portfolios and assignments with reflection built into them

Disincentives and penalties	Ensure that students know that poor performance in assessment can lead to failure	Do not condone behaviours that are considered to be unprofessional; ensure that standards are clear and that failure in assessment matters	Do not reward recall without evidence of ability to reflect
Participation	Encourage student representation on curriculum committees; student participation in determining content and process of teaching programme	Allow students to experience responsibility for shared learning (e.g. small group tasks, collaborative projects); encourage peer support, provide opportunities for realistic professional simulations (e.g. clinical practice improvement projects)	Foster discussion and debates on ethical and professional issues; provide opportunities for students to understand the values of others; provide opportunities to experience human diversity

Adapted from Gordon J. Fostering students' personal and professional development in medicine: a new framework for PPD. *Med Educ.* 2003; **37**: 341–9.[14]

The strength of this model lies in the fact that it is derived from research in the health policy field on factors that influence attitudes and behaviour, and as such it should translate to and be easily applied in the context of teaching, learning and assessing professionalism.

OUTCOME-BASED APPROACH

A wag once remarked that Columbus would have made a good medical educator. When he set off, he had no idea where he was going. When he arrived, he had no idea where he was. When he returned, he had no idea where he'd been! A basic educational tenet is that, ideally, learners need to know where they are going and how they will know when they get there. Outcome-based education is based on the simple notion that learning and teaching should be determined by *learning outcomes* rather than by a syllabus

– that is, it provides a model of learning that emphasises *what is expected* of learners, teachers, institutions, etc., rather than a prescription of what they should know.

A learning outcome here means the end point of a particular learning experience – something that can be defined, and ideally expressed in behavioural terms, so that it can be assessed. Outcomes give structure and direction to all concerned in the process, offer a clear indication of the type and depth of learning required to achieve them (or at least they compel educators to consider this) and provide a framework for assessment and evaluation. In theory, this should offer clarity and accountability, promote relevance, encourage self-directed learning and foster ownership. One outcome-based approach, which was first developed in Scotland and has since been adopted and adapted by a number of UK medical schools, and which has also been modified for use in postgraduate education, defines outcomes in three broad domains – 'What the doctor does', 'How the doctor approaches practice' and 'The doctor as a professional.'[15] More specific outcomes are defined within each domain. For example, 'The doctor as a professional' includes the outcomes 'An understanding of the roles of the doctor' and 'Acceptance of individual responsibility for self-care.' 'How the doctor approaches practice' includes 'Appropriate attitudes, ethical understanding and legal responsibilities.' These can then be defined at an appropriate level right down to that of an individual teaching session. Writing useful learning outcomes is not as easy as it may first appear. One simple approach is to aim for 'SMART' outcomes – that is, outcomes that are Specific, Measurable, Achievable, Relevant and Timed (i.e. given a timeline) – and these should be written, where possible, using 'action verbs.'[16]

In this respect, and particularly in the context of outcomes for professionalism education, a note of caution is necessary. John Hamilton, former Dean of the medical school in Newcastle, New South Wales, has argued that too much emphasis may be put on those outcomes that can be defined, possibly at the expense of those that cannot, excluding some of the more important areas of doctoring.[17] As Einstein is supposed to have said, 'Not all that can be counted counts, and not all that counts can be counted!' (indeed, if something *can* be counted it probably doesn't count in the first place!). However, outcomes should not be omitted simply because of their imprecision or aspirational intent. Outcomes in medical education must be wide in their scope, long in their timeline and deep in their relevance to professional development.[17]

LEARNING ENVIRONMENT

Also known as 'learning culture' or 'educational climate', the learning environment is the overall context and setting in which the learning and teaching are taking place. It is a complex entity, is multifactorial and operates on many levels, including the physical environment, how much learning is valued and supported, relationships between the institution, teachers and learners, and the emotional climate and support available. It is one of the most powerful influences on learning, so much so that one could argue that getting it right is not only a prerequisite for effective learning, but may also be half the battle – conversely, get it wrong and problems will arise. An environment that is conducive to learning is supportive and safe, fosters collaboration, values the contribution of individuals, and is based on mutual respect. Such an environment can be fostered and nurtured. Curriculum planners and teachers could do worse than invest time, energy and resources in this. Medical schools in the past have been likened to abusive family systems, with characteristic features of 'unrealistic expectations, denial, indirect communication patterns, rigidity and isolation.'[18] Although this analysis may seem unduly harsh, particularly in the light of the major reforms of the past decade, it allows insight into factors that may still stand in the way of providing an appropriate climate. Assessment is another aspect of the learning environment, is possibly the most important driver of learning (*see* Chapter 11), and the 'hidden curriculum' also operates through it (see below).

THE 'HIDDEN CURRICULUM'

In any learning situation there are at least four curricula in action – the *intended curriculum* (that is, the formal curriculum as articulated in stated learning outcomes, syllabuses, course materials, and so on), the *delivered curriculum*, or *curriculum in action* (this is largely ad hoc, informal and unscripted – what happens 'on the day'), the *assessed curriculum* (what is tested) and the *received curriculum* (that is, what the learners take away from the situation). An important component of the latter is the so-called 'hidden curriculum.' This was first described in the 1960s in primary education, and consists of the 'processes, pressures and constraints which fall outside … the formal curriculum, and which are often unarticulated and unexplored.'[19] It is the medium by which values and mores are transmitted, it operates at many levels (from an institutional level down to an individual learning situation), and is without doubt one of the most powerful and unrealised influences on professional development. It can either undermine or reinforce the formal curriculum – sadly often the former, the hidden messages effectively determining what the students see as the 'stuff' that matters, and explaining 'the mismatch between aims and outcomes in some aspects of medical training.'[20] For example, no matter how much a teacher exhorts learners to elicit patients' ideas, concerns and expectations in communication skills teaching, if students do not see this happening once they are on the wards or in the clinics, or worse still, they get the message that it is not important, they will soon stop bothering to do it. Similarly, if *their* ideas, concerns and expectations are not addressed, the teaching of this practice will be hollow and theoretical. This phenomenon has been well described and explored in undergraduate and postgraduate education, but less so in continuing medical education.[21] The hidden curriculum can be analysed in several ways – for example, by looking at institutional policies, assessment practices, and what has been called 'institutional slang.'[21] Examples from undergraduate education would include the increased value attached to research over teaching (institutional policy), greater emphasis on testing scientific knowledge than on attitudes (assessment practice), and reference to older patients as 'crumble' or labelling patients as 'difficult' or poor historians (institutional slang). The black humour that is characteristic of medical students and doctors also offers a window into the hidden curriculum.

A strategy for addressing the hidden or informal curriculum has been described at Indiana University School of Medicine.[22] Recognising the need for widespread cultural change, the initiative used an 'appreciative, narrative-based approach' (a method of organisational change originally used in community development), the aim being to align the informal curriculum with the formal one by promoting 'mindfulness on the part of every faculty member, resident, and staff member about the values we exhibit and thereby teach in our everyday interactions.'[22] A small team of volunteers (staff *and* students) conducted interviews with a range of individuals in the school, seeking stories about the best aspects of the informal curriculum and aspirations for change. These stories and emerging themes were fed back to school members, discussed and debated, and a process of change was initiated. Many instances of change have apparently been observed, ranging from self-reported changes in attitudes and behaviour, to modification of the selection process. The project is ongoing. There is clearly potential for this kind of approach to cultural change within organisations such as NHS trusts.

COMMUNICATION

The fundamental importance of good communication in clinical practice is beyond contention (*see* Chapter 5). However, formal education about communication at both undergraduate and postgraduate levels in the UK has until surprisingly recently been a 'minority activity', other than in GP vocational training. Historically it largely consisted of stand-alone courses, which despite innovative use of video, role play and simulated patients, were relatively ineffective. It was often not integrated with the core curriculum and, most importantly, skills were not assessed. For example, a survey of communication skills teaching in UK and Irish medical schools conducted in 1995–96 showed that although there had been progress since the last major survey in 1989, there was still considerable variability in course content, underpinning theory (or lack of it), degree of integration, duration and timing of teaching, and its assessment. Departments of general practice and psychiatry still predominated in delivering teaching, and there was variable involvement of non-medical disciplines (a diverse range of staff were involved, but there were concerns about capacity and maintaining skills). The main barriers to further development cited by respondents were lack of adequate physical resources and lack of suitably trained staff.[23]

BOX 10.5 KEY ELEMENTS OF PROPOSED CURRICULUM
FOR COMMUNICATION IN MEDICAL EDUCATION

Underlying philosophy
Communication teaching and learning:
- reflect the ethical principles of healthcare practice
- be evidence based
- enable learners to respond to individual patients' needs
- promote personal and professional development
- promote reflection.

Core competencies
These fall under the following broad headings:
- attitudes and values
- knowledge (including psychology of interpersonal communication)
- patient-centred consulting
- a set of core skills
- strategies for communication in specific circumstances (e.g. working with interpreters, breaking bad news)
- broad view of communication (i.e. not confined to doctor–patient interaction).

Adapted from Schofield T. A curriculum for communication in medical education. Appendix II. In: Macdonald E, editor. *Difficult Conversations in Medical Education*. Oxford: Oxford University Press; 2004.[23]

However, there has been a major expansion of communication skills teaching (CST) education in undergraduate education in the past decade (and to a much smaller extent, as yet, in postgraduate education), inspired partly by documents such as *Tomorrow's Doctors*, the report of the Bristol Inquiry,[24] and international consensus statements (the most recent of which was published in 1999).[25] A curriculum for communication in medical education has also been published, in which the underlying philosophy, a set of core competencies and approaches to learning and assessment are outlined[26] (*see* Box 10.5).

There is a rich and expanding research literature on communication and the doctor–patient relationship. Several frameworks that espouse the philosophy and principles described in the 'core curriculum' have been described, which are intended to guide teaching, practice *and* research. One that is rapidly becoming standard in the UK, at both undergraduate and postgraduate levels, is the Calgary–Cambridge framework.[27] This helps to promote a patient-centred approach since it is based on the so-called disease–illness model. The latter posits that in any doctor–patient encounter a search of two parallel frameworks is required, namely the *disease* framework (i.e. the symptoms, signs and other biomedical information needed to reach a differential, pathophysiological diagnosis) and the *illness* framework (i.e. the patient's unique experience, including ideas, concerns, feelings, and so on). Only by integrating the two frameworks can doctors achieve shared understanding of the patient's problem.

Using the Calgary–Cambridge framework (*see* Box 10.6), the process of communication can be broken down into units, and the component 'microskills' taught at an appropriate level.

BOX 10.6 A FRAMEWORK FOR COMMUNICATION SKILLS
TEACHING BASED ON THE CALGARY–CAMBRIDGE GUIDE[26]

Initiating the interview
- Establishing initial rapport
- Identifying the reason(s) for the consultation

Gathering information
- Exploration of the problem(s)
- Understanding the patient's perspective
- Providing structure for the consultation

Building the relationship
- Developing rapport
- Involving the patient

Explanation and planning
- Providing the correct amount and type of information
- Aiding accurate recall and understanding
- Achieving a shared understanding – incorporating the patient's perspective
- Planning – shared decision making

Closing the session
- Summarising
- 'Safety netting'

The need for a learner-centred approach that incorporates the educational principles described above is crucial. A 'mixed menu' of approaches involving practice and rehearsal with constructive feedback, use of simulation and role play, combining a skills-based approach with opportunities for reflection on attitudinal issues, is crucial.[28]

ETHICS AND THE LAW

The ability to evaluate ethical and legal issues raised by medical practice is a core clinical skill and a key attribute of professionalism. Various approaches to teaching ethics in higher education have been described[29] – for example, 'pragmatic', 'theoretical' and 'embedded.' With the pragmatic approach the starting point is the framework of rules, procedures and codes defined by regulating bodies. In theory this approach emphasises the relevance of ethics to everyday practice, but it tends to view regulation and raising of standards as a set of externally imposed constraints. The theoretical approach starts with the concepts and principles that underpin the codes of practice, together with the notions of professionalism and fitness to practise considered in the other two approaches. In theory this should lead to deeper understanding, although there is a danger that learners may fail to see its relevance and may marginalise the subject as being too theoretical. The embedded approach has ethics integrated into and taught within a broad programme in which students explore the nature of professionalism or the concept of 'fitness to practise.' Again this should promote relevance, but with a greater emphasis on autonomy, and individual responsibility for improving and maintaining standards. There is a place for all three approaches, although the embedded approach conforms most closely with the educational principles listed earlier.

As with communication, a core curriculum for ethics and medical law was proposed in a consensus statement published by UK teachers of ethics and law.[30] It argued that such teaching demands 'a balanced, sustained, academically rigorous and clinically relevant presentation of both ethics and the law in medicine, and of the relationship and tensions between them.'[30] It contended that ethics and law applied to medicine is an established academic discipline and should be introduced systematically, starting early on, and reinforced throughout the undergraduate course and beyond. It should be integrated with the core curriculum, should use a variety of teaching methods, should not be taught as an isolated subject, and must be formally assessed, both formatively and summatively. The list of areas to be covered is shown in Box 10.7. The authors of the consensus statement suggested that 'Many schools may wish to do more than we have outlined and this is to be commended. We believe that they should not do less.'[30]

BOX 10.7 CORE LIST OF ETHICS AND LEGAL TOPICS PROPOSED FOR UNDERGRADUATE EDUCATION

- Informed consent and refusal of treatment
- The clinical relationship – truthfulness, trust and communication
- Confidentiality and good clinical practice
- Medical research
- Human reproduction
- The 'new' genetics
- Children
- Mental disorders and disabilities
- Life, death, dying and killing
- Vulnerabilities created by the duties of doctors and medical students
- Resource allocation
- Rights

Source: Consensus Group of Teachers of Medical Ethics and Law in UK Medical Schools. Teaching medical ethics and law within medical education: a model for the UK core curriculum. *J Med Ethics*. 1998; **24**: 188–92.[30]

The overall aims of teaching and learning ethics should be to enable the learner to develop a coherent value system by reflecting on and thinking critically about ethical issues raised by contemporary medical practice. They should be able to revise this in the light of subsequent experience, identify the values underlying clinical decision making, and distinguish personal from professional and societal values. They should also understand the main professional obligations of doctors in the system in which they are working, distinguishing between ethical and legal duties, as well as recognise ethical dilemmas raised by the practice and study of medicine. They need to be familiar with the ethical concepts and principles that underpin good medical practice, to understand and appreciate alternative and sometimes competing approaches, and be able to argue and counter-argue, but ultimately to acknowledge the views of those with whom they disagree, and appreciate the strengths of those views. It is important to emphasise that ethical issues potentially arise in most clinical encounters, however mundane those issues may appear to be (e.g. how much information to give to a patient about the side-effects of medication), and that medical ethics is not *just* about 'the big issues' (e.g. related to new genetics, or end-of-life decisions).

Examples of 'embedded' ethics teaching from the case-led, integrated undergraduate curriculum at Newcastle University in the UK are shown in Box 10.8.

BOX 10.8 EXAMPLES OF 'EMBEDDED' ETHICS TEACHING SESSIONS FOR MEDICAL STUDENTS

First year: a lecture on 'ethics and the pharmaceutical industry' links with integrated teaching and learning focused around a case called 'The new drug' (other relevant areas covered are critical appraisal of pharmaceutical literature, including randomised controlled trials and drug adverts, and drug trials).

Second year: ethical issues related to resuscitation are explicitly highlighted and discussed in a clinical skills practical on CPR (and link with a small group session on end-of-life decisions, and other teaching about death and dying).

Third year: during a clinical rotation in infectious diseases an 'ethics and communication' session is dedicated to exploring ethical issues raised by HIV and AIDS, reflections on ethical dilemmas encountered by students in clinics during the rotation, and exploration of relevant communication issues using role play to develop negotiation and empathy skills (scenarios are contextualised in infectious diseases – for example, negotiating with a parent about not prescribing an antibiotic).

Fourth year: as part of a course on diagnostic medicine, a mock m negligence trial is held (focused on a case of a complicated head injury resulting in death of the patient), involving the contribution of practising lawyers acting as counsel for the claimant and defendant, and presided over by a judge.

Fifth year: a small group session explores aspects of medical error using clips from a TV documentary, case discussions and vignettes focused on patients' needs, and role play. Students are also asked to recall a recent mistake they may have made, or with which they have been directly involved, and to write a short description of what happened, followed by a discussion of responses to errors and how they might be prevented.

Acknowledgements are due to Reverend Bryan Vernon, Lecturer in Health Care Ethics, Newcastle University.

FOSTERING SELF-AWARENESS

Learning to be a doctor, and doctoring itself, may involve significant challenges to attitudes and values, preconceptions, motivation, self-esteem and well-being. At the same time, however well they have learned the science of medicine, doctors use themselves to practise 'the art.' This requires a considerable degree of self-awareness – 'insight into how one's life experiences and emotional make-up affect one's interactions with patients, families and other professionals.'[31] Historically, basic training and CPD programmes have paid scant attention to promotion of self-awareness and provision of support. This may have contributed to the well recognised increase in cynicism and decline in empathy noted as students progress through training and into professional practice. For example, certain dysfunctional beliefs – such as the idea that limitations in knowledge represent a personal failing, or that to be truly 'professional' means keeping one's uncertainties and emotions to oneself – may affect patient care.

Several authors have suggested that curricula (both undergraduate and postgraduate) should explicitly address enhancement of self-awareness. There is some evidence, albeit limited, showing a correlation between students' self-awareness and both patient-centredness and increased sense of professional responsibility.[32]

One model proposed by the American Academy on Physician and Patient consists of four core elements – physicians' attitudes and beliefs, challenging clinical situations, physicians' feelings and emotions, and self-care (*see* Box 10.9) – all of which are dependent on reflection and discussion, ideally in supportive groups.[31]

BOX 10.9 A CORE CURRICULUM FOR
PHYSICIAN PERSONAL AWARENESS[31]

Physicians' beliefs and attitudes
- Core beliefs, personal philosophy
- Influences of family of origin
- Gender issues
- Socio-cultural issues

Physicians' feelings and emotional responses in patient care
- Love, caring, attraction and boundary setting in medical care
- Conflict and anger

Challenging clinical situations
- 'Difficult patients'
- Caring for dying patients
- Medical mistakes

Physician self-care
- Balancing personal and professional lives
- Preventing and managing stress/burnout/impairment

THE ROLE OF HUMANITIES, CREATIVE WRITING AND NARRATIVE APPROACHES

A strong argument has been made for introducing humanities into both undergraduate and postgraduate curricula to help learners to develop 'a more compassionate understanding of the individual in society, to inspire empathy with patients and colleagues, and to become more "rounded" people themselves.'[33] The idea is that the study of poetry, prose or drama, painting or other art forms will foster development of self-awareness, and will help learners to achieve a better understanding of the nature of suffering and the 'illness experience', as well as helping them to hone important skills such as observation, critical analysis and reflection. In addition, it may help them to recognise how factors such as culture, gender, sexual orientation, social status, education and personality (to name just a few) influence health and illness and the doctor–patient relationship. All in all, the study of humanities, it is argued, should equip the learner with a toolkit with which to analyse and understand the issues that confront them in their daily practice.

Medical teachers have probably always used literary and other references in their teaching, either to illustrate important points or to spice up the subject. Specific medical humanities programmes first started to appear in the 1970s, and the trend has gained considerable momentum in the past decade. In a recent survey, for example, three-quarters of American medical schools reported that humanities were included in their curricula. There is at least one dedicated journal (Medical Humanities edition of the *Journal of Medical Ethics*), and two leading international medical education journals (*Medical Education* and *Academic Medicine*) have dedicated humanities sections. There is also a steady output of useful 'how to do it' books, articles, and online resources.[34-36] One approach to using medical humanities is shown in Box 10.10.

BOX 10.10 ONE APPROACH TO TEACHING ABOUT
PROFESSIONALISM USING HUMANITIES

A structure for a session using an arts resource (e.g. a piece of prose, an extract of a play or a poem):

- *Have a clear aim* (not only an educational aim, but why this is the best approach).
- *Find and select a resource* (considering its relevance to personal and professional development).
- *Design appropriate exercise(s)* (ideally ones that spark further creativity).
- *Achieve engagement with the learners* (including paying attention to the setting).
- *Facilitate responses* (e.g. picking up cues from learners' responses and interpreting and developing ideas).
- *Contextualise* (i.e. explore relevance to everyday life and practice).

Adapted from Powley E, Higson R. *The Arts in Medical Education. A practical guide.* Oxford: Radcliffe Publishing; 2005.[34]

As with ethics and other subjects, use of humanities is likely to be most effective when integrated into the core curriculum. Indeed, if it is taught as a stand-alone subject (either as a separate course, or as an elective or optional component) it is likely to be seen by many learners as irrelevant and a waste of precious time and energy (after all, there are important facts to be learned out there!). Teaching should be underpinned by the key educational principles outlined earlier, and as one set of authors put it, 'We believe the aim should be to involve students emotionally, to stimulate the right brain, and encourage self-reflection. If one subscribes to this view, then didacticism, lecturing from notes or focussing too much on theory is counter-productive.'[37]

The introduction of arts and humanities into postgraduate education has lagged behind undergraduate education, yet it may be even more important for established practitioners to have opportunities to explore broader dimensions of their work, not least in the 'brave new world' of increasing regulation, managed care, and so on. There may be benefits, not only for patients in terms of more holistic care, but also for the professionals themselves – for example, preventing 'burnout', helping to achieve a healthy work–life balance, and perhaps re-energising their practice. In fact this area is beginning to receive attention, with dedicated sections in mainstream journals, descriptions of educational interventions, and suggestions for incorporating humanities into postgraduate training and continuing professional development.

A beautifully crafted piece of prose, an unusual painting or a movie clip may act as a potent stimulus to reflection and discussion. However, just as powerful an approach, and possibly more so, may be provided by reflection upon something written by health professionals themselves. Creative writing is an approach to professional development that has emerged in the last decade.[38] The aim is not to write a publishable masterpiece, and creative writing workshops do not require literary skill. In theory, the combination of writing followed by open discussion with peers in a safe setting should lead to critical and reflective examination of professional practice, and help people to deal with uncertainty and confront uncomfortable emotions. Creative writing workshops and groups are generally very positively evaluated, and offer an approach that could be applied in virtually any learning situation.

Related to this, narrative approaches have also found a place in medicine in the last few years. One activity that is universal to all cultures and social groups, so far as we know, is storytelling. Historically, this has served a variety of functions, acting as a means whereby our myths and legends, values, customs and social mores, and ways of seeing and behaving, have been communicated within and between generations. Stories, or narratives, provide social cohesion, separating 'us' from 'others', and helping to give meaning to our lives, and to help us to create order out of chaos. Furthermore, we are continually engaged in a process of recreating or reconstructing our own narratives – a lifelong process which enables us to make sense of the world and to process new experiences. To quote one author on the subject, we 'dream in narrative, daydream in narrative, remember, anticipate, hope, despair, believe, doubt, plan, revise, criticise, construct, gossip, learn, hate and love by narrative.'[39]

Health professionals experience their work within a narrative framework which shapes and gives meaning to what they are feeling, defining how, why and in what way they act, and to a great extent how those around them respond to and interact with them. Thus understanding narrative may provide helpful insights for health professionals in a range of areas, enabling us to adopt a more holistic approach to care provision, and to better understand both the patient's perspective and our own.

INVOLVING PATIENTS

Sir William Osler's dictum that 'it is a safe rule to have no teaching without a patient for a text, and the best teaching is that taught by the patient himself' is well known. The importance of learning from the patient has been emphasised to generations of medical students, who have been exhorted to 'Listen to the patient – he is telling you the diagnosis', and suchlike. Yet their role has been largely passive, the patient acting as interesting teaching material, but little more than a medium through which the teacher teaches. However, there is a growing literature on the potential contribution that patients can make to education and training of health professionals, over and above being simply (and passively) an 'interesting case'.[40] Patients can not only recount the stories of their illnesses (which are quite different from the medical histories that the student or doctor *take*), providing deeper and broader insights into their problems, but they can also give feedback to both teachers and learners, not least about aspects of their professionalism. Some patients in fact see themselves as having a distinct, pro-active teaching role, and 'expert patients' are being increasingly involved in medical education at both undergraduate and postgraduate levels, either directly in teaching or to inform curriculum development (e.g. in crafting roles for simulated patients). There is also a rapidly expanding literature documenting patient illness narratives in a host of clinical areas, especially cancer, and dedicated websites such as the DIPEX (Database of Personal Experience of Health and Illness) website,[41] all of which are potentially rich sources of educational material. Moreover, in November 2005 an international conference entitled 'Where's the patient voice in health professional education?' was held in Vancouver as a means of exploring the many ways in which patients may be involved in learning and teaching activities.[42]

Although a small amount of early patient contact has been a feature of traditional medical curricula for several decades, it has only been seen as a crucial component of a doctor's training in the last decade or so. A recent systematic review of the literature on early contact found that, despite methodological weaknesses in most of the studies, there was good evidence that such experience fostered self-awareness, motivated learners, and helped them to develop a professional identity. Most importantly, it helped to foster empathy towards ill people, helped learners to understand professional roles and responsibilities, and orientated them to the health needs of populations.[43]

INTERPROFESSIONAL EDUCATION (IPE) AND LEARNING

We know that effective teamwork leads to improved outcomes and better quality of care for patients. However, health professionals have generally been ill-prepared by their education for working in the multidisciplinary environments that are increasingly the norm in healthcare. Professional 'tribalism' is perpetuated by a host of factors, not least ignorance about roles, negative stereotypes and conflicts of interest.

Interprofessional education – defined as 'occurring when two or more professions learn with, from and about each other to facilitate collaboration in practice'[44] – is one of the major educational trends of the time. Common learning programmes have been encouraged at pre-registration level, and CPD is increasingly team based. Advocates of IPE claim that this will lead to better collaboration and teamwork, ultimately for the benefit of patients. Although the jury is still out as to whether or not these aims have been achieved, evidence about the efficacy of various approaches is beginning to emerge. In a best-evidence medical education (BEME) systematic review of evaluations of IPE,[45] the authors call for the adoption of a common outcomes model for measuring the 'products' of IPE to allow better comparisons between studies. They conclude that more evaluations are needed and that many unanswered questions remain about IPE. However, IPE certainly has a powerful intuitive appeal. Professional attributes appear to be generic, and the case for a core curriculum for all heathcare students focused on the development of 'inter-professionalism' has been made.[46]

PATIENT SAFETY

Medical errors are common and inevitable, especially given the increasingly complex nature of healthcare. However, although they recognise both the inevitability of error and the fact that most mistakes are due as much to systems rather than to individual failure, doctors have difficulty dealing with error when it occurs. An extensive literature has identified the nature and scale of the problem, underlying concepts and theories, and how error might be prevented, yet there is still a high incidence of mistakes and 'near misses.' Lucian Leape, paediatric surgeon and health policy analyst at Harvard, has argued that 'the most fundamental change that will be needed if [medicine is] to make meaningful progress in error reduction is a cultural one'[47] – that is, health professionals must accept that error is inevitable, even when the highest standards are set. Historically, students are socialised to strive for error-free practice. There is a major emphasis on perfection, and mistakes are seen as unacceptable and therefore judged as failures of character when they occur.[48] Furthermore, the nature of 'being responsible' for patients' welfare means that, paradoxically, when something goes wrong it must be the doctor's responsibility – a situation that is fuelled by an apparently increasingly litigious society. It appears to be difficult for a doctor to say 'sorry' – a basic act of compassion – because this may be construed as an admission of guilt, yet the emotional impact of error upon the doctor may be profound. Dealing with such issues in the education and training of health professionals is one important component of strategies to change the culture. Thus 'patient safety' has emerged over the past few years as an important and discrete element of medical education at both undergraduate and postgraduate levels. Box 10.11 shows a list of topics that could be included in a patient safety curriculum.

BOX 10.11 POTENTIAL TOPICS FOR A PATIENT SAFETY CURRICULUM

- *Overview and context* (overview of the problem; society's changing expectations; professionalism and the 'culture' of medicine; codes of practice such as *Good Medical Practice*).
- *Nature and scale of the problem* (the 'epidemiology' of error, adverse events and 'near misses').
- *Underlying concepts and theories* (taxonomy of error; systems versus individual; Human Factor research; 'Swiss cheese' and other models; iceberg concept; approaches to prevention).
- *Learning from others* (the aviation and other 'high-risk' industries; models of good practice within medicine, e.g. anaesthetics).
- *Responding to error – the individual* (impact on patients, carers and health professionals).
- *Responding to error – systems, organisations and policy* (clinical governance; policy initiatives, including national standards, NPSA, Medicines Control and Medical Devices Agencies; adverse-incident-reporting systems; root cause analysis and other approaches).
- *Communication issues* (patient-centred model; communicating about risk and benefit; disclosure of error and dealing with the response).
- *Ethical and legal issues* (individual versus collective responsibility; truth telling; whistleblowing; the legal context).

- *Errors in procedures* (what common errors occur with procedures, including devices, and how they come about; how they might be prevented).
- *Errors in prescribing* (what common errors occur with prescribing, and how they come about; how they might be prevented).
- *Errors in clinical reasoning* (what common errors occur with clinical reasoning, including diagnosis and management, and how they come about; how they might be prevented).
- *The healthcare team and error* (different perspectives on error; inter-professional communication; communication within the team).
- *Involving patients* (models of involving patients in decision making; communicating about risk and benefits).

In the UK, the National Patient Safety Agency (NPSA), established in 2001, has adopted an educational approach to disseminating good practice, including a nationwide training programme for junior doctors and funding for several medical schools to develop relevant teaching materials.[49] Similar educational strategies have been implemented in other countries, such as the USA and Australia.[49]

PERSONAL DEVELOPMENT PLANS, APPRAISAL AND REVALIDATION

Personal development plans are becoming the norm throughout the educational continuum, to guide personal *and* professional development in both formative and summative contexts – for example, in continuing professional development,[50] often forming part of a learning portfolio (*see* Chapter 11). At the time of writing, a major consultation exercise is under way in the UK in response to a report by the Chief Medical Officer, Liam Donaldson, entitled *Good Doctors, Safer Patients*.[51] This consists of proposals to strengthen the system of assuring and improving doctors' performance and to protect the safety of patients, including appraisal and revalidation.

THE LEARNER'S PERSPECTIVE

One of the problems in designing and delivering a professionalism curriculum is potential resistance from learners. In the UK, it is still the case that the majority of students who enter medicine come from a science background. The 'hidden curriculum' messages about what knowledge is valued still favour scientific and clinical knowledge over more 'touchy-feely' areas (which, in any case, are only 'common sense'!). Furthermore, it has long been recognised that medical students seem to become more cynical as they progress through their training, with an associated decline in empathy.[52] How to 'stop the rot' is a challenge for medical educators.[53] It is clearly crucial that learners can see the relevance and are motivated, and adherence to the educational principles outlined earlier in this chapter should in theory help this. Involving learners in the development and implementation of teaching about professionalism may also help. In a thought-provoking article, a medical student from Indiana State Medical School offered 'three easy steps' for clinical educators to effect change.[54] First, 'be the lesson you want the students to take away', emphasising the fundamental importance of role modelling and the hidden curriculum. Secondly, create and nurture a sense of 'community' by showing respect for students and developing a rapport with them, which will foster the third element, good communication.[54] Obvious analogies can be drawn here between teacher–student and doctor–patient relationships.

It is important to consider the issue of maturity of the learner. Hilton and Slotnick argued that professionalism is an acquired state (as opposed to a trait), and suggested an early phase of 'proto-professionalism.' Professionalism is only realised through experience and reflection on experience, and that 'adverse environmental conditions in the hidden curriculum may have powerful attritional effects.'[55] Hilton and Slotnick suggested several elements of education and training pertinent to the development of professionalism that they felt were currently *under*-emphasised in curricula. These included art, humanism, reflection, mindfulness, generalism, collegiality and inter-professionalism. More recently, Jill Gordon of Sydney has highlighted the need to ensure that learners have opportunities to 'work in teams, to develop skills in respectful but assertive communication and to practise averting error in a blame-free environment.'[56]

Finally, one of the most potent ways of ensuring that teaching and learning about professionalism is taken seriously by students is to assess it. This is explored further in Chapter 11.

CONCLUSIONS

At the time of writing, inclusion of education about professionalism in medical curricula is without doubt 'an idea whose time has come.'[57] However, according to the result of a recent survey of UK medical schools conducted by researchers from King's College London, there is still some way to go.[58] For example, they found that although the consensus was that recent curriculum reform had brought about major improvement, it appeared that some of the negative effects of the hidden curriculum were still prevalent, considered by many to be the biggest threat to development of appropriate professional attitudes and behaviour. Success appeared to depend upon creating and maintaining a positive learning culture.

REFERENCES

1 Flexner A. *Medical Education. A comparative study.* New York: Macmillan Company; 1925. p. 226.

2 McManus IC, Powis DA, Wakeford R *et al.* Intellectual aptitude tests and A-levels for selecting UK school leaver entrants for medical school. *BMJ.* 2005; **331**: 555–9.

3 Stephenson A, Higgs R, Sugarman J. Teaching professional development in medical schools. *Lancet.* 2001; **357**: 867–70.

4 Cruess SR, Cruess SL. Professionalism must be taught. *BMJ.* 1997; **315**: 1674–5.

5 General Medical Council. *Tomorrow's Doctors. Recommendations on undergraduate medical education.* London: General Medical Council; 1993.

6 General Medical Council. *Tomorrow's Doctors.* London: General Medical Council; 2003.

7 General Medical Council. *Good Medical Practice.* London: General Medical Council; 1995.

8 www.gmc-uk.org/guidance/good_medical_practice/index.asp (accessed May 2008).

9 American Board of Internal Medicine. *Project Professionalism.* Philadelphia, PA: American Board of Internal Medicine; 1994.

10 www.foundationprogramme.nhs.uk/pages/home/key-documents#foundation-program-curriculum (accessed May 2008).

11 http://rcpsc.medical.org/canmeds/index.php (accessed May 2008).

12 Chastonay P, Brenner E, Peel S *et al.* The need for more efficacy and relevance in medical education. *Med Educ.* 1996; **30**: 235–8.

13 Howe A. Twelve tips for developing professional attitudes in training. *Med Teach.* 2003; **25**: 485–7.

14 Gordon J. Fostering students' personal and professional development in medicine: a new framework for PPD. *Med Educ.* 2003; **37**: 341–9.

15 Harden RM, Crosby JR, Davis MH. An introduction to outcome-based education. *Med Teach.* 1999; **21**: 7–14.

16 Spencer J, Jordan R. Educational outcomes and leadership to meet the needs of modern health care. *Qual Health Care.* 2001; **10**: ii38–45.

17 Hamilton JD. Outcomes in medical education must be wide, long and deep. *Med Teach.* 1999; **21**: 125–6.

18 McKegney CP. Medical education: a neglectful and abusive family system. *Fam Med.* 1989; **21**: 452–7.

19 Cribb A, Bignold S. Towards the reflexive medical school: the hidden curriculum and medical education research. *Stud Higher Educ.* 1999; **24**: 195–209.

20 Howe A. Professional development in undergraduate medical curricula – the key to the door of a new culture? *Med Educ.* 2002; **36**: 353–9.

21 Bennett N, Lockyer J, Mann K *et al.* Hidden curriculum in continuing medical education. *J Contin Educ Health Prof.* 2004; **24**: 145–52.

22 Suchman AL, Williamson PR, Litzelman DK *et al.* and the Relationship-Centred

Care Initiative Discovery Team. Toward an informal curriculum that teaches professionalism: transforming the social environment of a medical school. *J Gen Intern Med.* 2004; **19:** 501–4.

23 Hargie O, Dickson D, Boohan M *et al.* A survey of communication skills training in UK Schools of Medicine: present practices and prospective proposals. *Med Teach.* 1998; **32:** 25–34.

24 www.bristol-inquiry.org.uk/final_report (accessed May 2008).

25 Makoul G, Schofield T. Communication teaching and assessment in medical education: an international consensus statement. *Patient Educ Counsel.* 1999; **137:** 191–5.

26 Schofield T. Appendix II. A curriculum for communication in medical education. In: Macdonald E, editor. *Difficult Conversations in Medicine.* Oxford: Oxford University Press; 2004.

27 Silverman J, Kurtz S, Draper J. *Skills for Communicating with Patients.* 2nd ed. Oxford: Radcliffe Publishing; 2005.

28 Kurtz S, Silverman J, Draper J. *Teaching and Learning Communication in Medicine.* 2nd ed. Oxford: Radcliffe Publishing; 2005.

29 Philosophical and Religious Studies Subject Centre Learning and Teaching Support Network. *Approaches to Ethics in Higher Education: teaching ethics across the core curriculum.* Leeds: Philosophical and Religious Studies Subject Centre Learning and Teaching Support Network; 2004.

30 Consensus Group of Teachers of Medical Ethics and Law in UK Medical Schools. Teaching medical ethics and law within medical education: a model for the UK core curriculum. *J Med Ethics.* 1998; **24:** 188–92.

31 Novack DH, Suchman AL, Clark W *et al.* Calibrating the physician: personal awareness and effective patient care. *JAMA.* 1997; **278:** 502–9.

32 Bennbassat J, Baumal R. Enhancing self-awareness in medical students: an overview of teaching approaches. *Acad Med.* 2005; **80:** 156–61.

33 Philipp R, Baum M, Mawson A *et al. Humanities in Medicine: beyond the millennium.* London: Nuffield Trust; 1999.

34 Powley E, Higson R. *The Arts in Medical Education: a practical guide.* Oxford: Radcliffe Publishing; 2005.

35 Alexander M, Lenahan P, Pavlov A, editors. *Cinemeducation: a comprehensive guide to using film in medical education.* Oxford: Radcliffe Publishing; 2005.

36 http://medhum.med.nyu.edu/syllabi.html (accessed May 2008).

37 Wetzel P, Hinchey J, Verghese A. The teaching of medical humanities. *Clin Teach.* 2005; **2:** 91–6.

38 Bolton G. *Reflective Practice: writing and professional development.* London: Paul Chapman Publishing; 2001.

39 Greenhalgh T, Hurwitz B. Narrative-based medicine: why study narrative? *BMJ.* 1999; **318:** 48–50.

40 Spencer J *et al.* Patient-oriented learning: a review of the role of the patient in the education of medical students. *Med Educ.* 2000; **34:** 851–7.

41 www.dipex.org/DesktopDefault.aspx (accessed May 2008).

42 www.health-disciplines.ubc.ca/DHCC/PtsVoiceReportBook.pdf (accessed May 2008).

43 Littlewood S, Ypinazar V, Margolis SA *et al.* Early practical experience and the social responsiveness of clinical education: systematic review. *BMJ.* 2005; **331:** 387–91.

44 Barr H. *Interprofessional Education, 1997–2000: a review.* London: UK Centre for Advancement of Inter-Professional Education (CAIPE); 2000.

45 Hammick M, Freeth D, Koppel I *et al.* A best evidence systematic review of interprofessional education. *Med Teach.* 2007; **29**: 735–51.

46 McNair RP. The case for educating health care students in professionalism as the core content of interprofessional education. *Med Educ.* 2005; **39**: 456–64.

47 Leape LL. Error in medicine. *JAMA.* 1994; **272**: 1851–7.

48 Lester H, Tritter Q. Medical error: a discussion of the medical construction of error and suggestions for reforms of medical education to decrease error. *Med Educ.* 2001; **35**: 855–61.

49 www.npsa.nhs.uk/health (accessed May 2008).

50 www.patient.co.uk/showdoc/40002441/ (accessed May 2008).

51 www.dh.gov.uk/en/PublicationsandStatistics/Publications/PublicationsPolicy AndGuidelines/DH_9137232 (accessed May 2008).

52 Spiro H, McCrea Cumen MG, Peschel E *et al. Empathy and the Practice of Medicine: beyond the pill and the scalpel.* New Haven, CT: Yale University Press; 1993.

53 Spencer J. Decline in empathy in medical education: how can we stop the rot? *Med Educ.* 2004; **38**: 916–17.

54 Skiles J. Teaching professionalism: a medical student's opinion. *Clin Teach.* 2005; **2**: 66–71.

55 Hilton SR, Slotnick HB. Proto-professionalism: how professionalisation occurs across the continuum of medical education. *Med Educ.* 2005; **39**: 58–65.

56 Gordon J. Progressing professionalism. *Med Educ.* 2006; **40**: 936–8.

57 www.quotedb.com/quotes/147 (accessed May 2008).

58 Stephenson AE, Adshead LE, Higgs RH. The teaching of professional attitudes within UK medical schools: reported difficulties and good practice. *Med Educ.* 2006; **40**: 1072–80.

CHAPTER 11

Assessing professionalism

This chapter explores:

- the purposes of assessment
- basic concepts in assessment
- the utility of assessment
- the ideal instrument for assessment of professionalism
- what the literature says about assessment of professionalism
- workplace-based assessment
- self-assessment and reflection
- the use of portfolios
- assessing communication
- peer assessment
- unprofessional conduct – lapses of professional behaviour.

> Although assessing professionalism poses many challenges, gauging and ascertaining growth in professionalism is impossible without measurement.
>
> *Lynch et al., 2004*[1]

INTRODUCTION

As we have seen, professionalism is a complex and dynamic concept that is influenced by a wide range of factors. Interest in the assessment of professionalism has grown in the past decade, mirroring the increased focus on learning and teaching professionalism – but the challenges are formidable. However, by shying away from these challenges the medical profession sends the wrong message to the public, and is ultimately doing a disservice to society, students and practitioners alike.[2,3] The greatest challenge has been the absence of a set of measurement instruments, although at the time of writing a huge 'industry' is engaged in developing and testing appropriate approaches and tools, some of which will be discussed in this chapter. Other difficulties include defining and describing those elements of professionalism that we wish (or need) to measure, ensuring that observations of behaviour are representative, and defining relevant situations and settings in which measurement – including observations of *lapses* in professional behaviour (see below) – should take place.[2] What tends to be assessed is observed 'professional' behaviours, while other aspects of professionalism are ignored.

WHY ASSESS?

It is impossible to overstate the importance of assessment (or evaluation, as it is more commonly called in North America), not least because it is recognised as an important driver of learning. In fact, assessment serves many potential purposes (*see* Box 11.1), often more than one at the same time. It can also have a number of undesirable consequences – for example, driving learning in an inappropriate direction, creating a hurdle-jump, 'pass and forget' mentality through concentration only on surface learning, loss of self-esteem and humiliation among those who are judged as being not 'up to standard', engendering unhelpful, possibly unhealthy and probably undesirable competitiveness, and adversely affecting progress and/or influencing career decisions.

BOX 11.1 PURPOSES OF ASSESSMENT IN MEDICAL/ CLINICAL EDUCATION AND TRAINING

- Measuring academic achievement.
- Certifying competence.
- Assuring standards (e.g. that an individual meets predetermined minimal standards).
- Diagnosing problems.
- Encouraging appropriate learning (what, how and when).
- Providing motivation and direction.
- Evaluating of teacher or course effectiveness.
- Predicting future performance.
- Discriminating between candidates (e.g. for entry to specialist training programmes).

Historically, the sensible and rational use of assessment in medical education and training has been bedevilled by conservative, even intransigent attitudes, leading one author to refer to the 'PHOG' that seems to descend when otherwise erudite academics sit down to discuss issues such as assessment (where PHOG stands for **Prejudice, Hunch, Opinion and Guesswork!**[4]). In the past, assessment has tended to be seen as a necessary evil, often only considered as an afterthought, and added as a 'bolt-on' extra to an educational programme, often leading to a degree of mal-alignment within the curriculum between teaching and assessment. A vast literature now exists about many aspects of assessment in medical education (indeed there are international conferences dedicated to the subject), yet little reference may be made by curriculum committees or course planners to the formidable evidence base that has accumulated, resulting in the use of inappropriate instruments, not least in the area of assessment of professionalism.

UTILITY OF ASSESSMENT

Cees van der Vleuten of Maastricht Medical School proposed a helpful way of looking at the properties of an assessment instrument in which the 'utility' or usefulness of the instrument is seen as a function of the relationship between several elements.[5] These are the instrument's validity and reliability, its effects on learning (its educational impact), its acceptability (to *all* stakeholders), and an inverse relationship with cost (including human resource costs) (*see* Box 11.2).

BOX 11.2 UTILITY OF AN ASSESSMENT INSTRUMENT (AFTER VAN DER VLEUTEN[5])

Utility $= V \times R \times EI \times A \times F$
where:
V $=$ validity (*see* Box 11.3 for explanation)
R $=$ reliability (*see* Box 11.3 for explanation)
EI $=$ educational impact
A $=$ acceptability
F $=$ feasibility (of which cost is an important element)

As with any specialist subject, assessment has its own jargon, which can be confusing and is often misunderstood. Definitions of some of the more commonly used terms are listed in Box 11.3.

Over the past 20 years, research into assessment in medicine has been dominated by a psychometric and thus predominantly quantitative and statistical approach, with a major focus on reliability and generalisability.[6] This has been achieved by building in standardisation and structure (a good example is the Objective Structured Clinical Examination, or OSCE), arguably at the expense of validity. Although reliability is clearly an extremely important dimension of assessment, more recently there has been a move towards approaches that are more qualitative and which feel more authentic,[6,7] prompted to a large extent by efforts to assess professionalism.

In practice, of course, there is usually some kind of trade-off between the elements of utility. For example, true/false-type multiple-choice questions as a test of knowledge are highly reliable (one can sample widely across a subject area), are acceptable, and of course are cheap (scripts can be marked by computer). However, their validity may be questionable, in that they often only test knowledge at the level of recall, and their influence on learning may be to encourage rote learning and cramming. On the other hand, the traditional long case clinical examination has considerable validity (real patient with a real problem), drives learning in an appropriate direction and is thus widely accepted, but its reliability is poor (because it is based on a single case – clinical competencies are highly content-specific) and its cost is high.[8]

BOX 11.3 BASIC CONCEPTS IN ASSESSMENT

Formative and summative assessment
- Formative assessment – this addresses the question 'How are you doing?', the main purpose being to provide learners with feedback about their progress and to guide further development.
- Summative assessment – this addresses the question 'How have you done?', the main aim being to make a decision about attainment, progress or fitness to practise. Summative assessments also have a formative effect, whether intended or not.

Validity
- Face validity – whether or not the instrument appears to measure what it is supposed to measure and/or what we think it is measuring.
- Construct validity – whether the instrument actually measures the theoretical construct that underpins what is being measured, ideally judged against a gold standard.
- Content validity – whether the instrument samples sufficiently the

key components or 'domains' of the construct being measured (i.e. representative, enough times).
- Consequential/predictive validity – whether the instrument can predict future behaviour.
- Criterion validity – how well the instrument correlates with other measures of what is being assessed.

Reliability

This is the extent to which the instrument consistently measures what it is supposed to measure.
- Internal reliability/consistency – a measure of whether the instrument is assessing one concept/construct, and whether scores on individual items would be correlated with scores on all other items.
- Stability – an assessment of the ability of the instrument to produce similar results when applied by different observers (*inter*-rater reliability) or by the same observer on different occasions (*intra*-rater reliability).
- Test–retest reliability – whether the instrument produces the same result if used on the same sample on two separate occasions.

Competence and performance
- Competence – how someone behaves under test conditions.
- Performance – how someone behaves in everyday practice.

(Note that a gap between 'competence' and 'performance' has been well documented.)

REQUIREMENTS FOR ASSESSMENT OF PROFESSIONALISM

As discussed in earlier chapters, if we accept that 'professionalism' consists of a complex combination of attributes, incorporating both behaviours and attitudes, and is both developmental and context-dependent, what important features should we look for in any assessment instruments? With reference to van der Vleuten's utility equation (*see* Box 11.2), we would obviously want them to be reliable, valid, acceptable, feasible and cost-effective, and to drive learning appropriately. For authenticity's sake we might prefer assessment to be undertaken as much as possible in the workplace. It has also been argued that a useful situation in which to assess professionalism is when there is some kind of values conflict[2,3] (e.g. when a learner is asked to do something, such as perform an intimate examination of a patient under anaesthetic, which conflicts with their own values and/or codes of practice). Thus an instrument should take account of how these conflicts are resolved. Since much of professional practice involves working with others in a team, seeking the views of colleagues could enhance judgements about an individual's professionalism, as could soliciting the views of patients. Given that assessment invariably involves sampling behaviour, we would wish to make sure that enough appropriate relevant events or situations are sampled. Finally, recognising the importance of reflection in both daily practice and professional development, we might want to look at an individual's reflective behaviour, in particular what was learned during clinical experience and, following critical incidents, why a lapse in professional behaviour might have occurred, and what and how the person changed as a result. Some of these issues will be considered in this chapter after the following exploration of what the literature has to say about the assessment of professionalism.

WHAT THE LITERATURE SAYS ABOUT THE ASSESSMENT OF PROFESSIONALISM

Several major review articles and a book about assessment of professionalism have recently been published. Arnold reviewed over 170 papers from a 30-year period,[9] classifying assessment instruments into three groups, namely those addressing professionalism as part of general clinical competence, those approaching professionalism as a single construct, and those addressing separate elements of professionalism such as humanism or ethical reasoning. Her main conclusions were that there was a need to develop rigorous qualitative methods, to strengthen quantitative approaches and to focus on behaviours that highlight how value conflicts are resolved, while taking account of the context in which professional behaviours and lapses occur. Lynch and colleagues reviewed 191 articles published between 1982 and 2002, reporting the use of 88 instruments.[1] Of these, 49 studies looked at ethical reasoning, and 27 were described as 'comprehensive' (i.e. they attempted to measure two or more elements of professionalism). However, most were based on self-assessment (see below) and delayed recall, and very few were designed for use over time. There was also great variability in the extent to which reliability and validity were examined and reported in the studies. The main recommendation was the need to develop more performance-based and longitudinal assessments.

Veloski and colleagues conducted a systematic review of papers published between 1984 and 2002, using a panel of 12 national experts in the USA, and identified a total of 134 empirical studies related to the concept of professionalism.[10] Again the majority of the studies looked at specific components of professionalism (mainly ethical or moral reasoning), with many instruments assessing the learning environment or group behaviour rather than individual behaviour, and only a few addressing professionalism as a comprehensive construct. The authors' conclusion was that there were 'few well documented studies that can be used to measure professionalism formatively or summatively'.[10] Ginsburg and colleagues also reviewed the literature in 2000 and offered a number of observations.[3] First, methods that depend on an abstract and idealised concept, such as 'professionalism', focus attention on *people* rather than on *behaviour*, the underlying assumption being that it is a set of stable attributes (further ignoring the fact that these attributes and traits are only weakly predictive of a person's later behaviour). Secondly, behaviour may be a manifestation of attempts to resolve a conflict between two equally valid or competing values. As mentioned above, of particular relevance here is *how* the conflict is resolved – the process of resolution is of as much interest and relevance as the outcome. Thirdly, it seems, historically, that assessors have been generally reluctant to pass judgement on individuals about relatively *minor* lapses in behaviour (as opposed to clearly aberrant behaviour). Finally, the authors pointed out that professional behaviour is highly context-dependent. As they put it, 'One can imagine a basically honest person lying to a patient given a particular context. This does not automatically mean that the person is dishonest, and therefore unprofessional. Certainly in social situations, a decision to always tell the full truth would be considered highly inappropriate.'[3] Clearly, methods of assessment need to take account of these grey (and not insignificant) areas.

Epstein and Hundert reviewed 195 papers in 2002, identifying a wide range of assessment tools, including many innovative approaches.[11] They found that few of the reported methods relied on observations in real-life situations, incorporated the views of either peers or patients, or used measures that predicted clinical outcomes. They recommended continuing development and refinement of new formats, including the assessment of areas such as management of uncertainty and teamwork, but argued that development of any programme of professionalism assessment must be backed up by appropriate support and mentoring systems.

A book on measurement of professionalism edited by David Stern,[2] published in 2005, explores a wide range of aspects, including the interaction of ethics, law and professionalism, assessment of moral reasoning, measurement of empathy, teamwork and lifelong learning, peer assessment, use of portfolios, student selection, professional accreditation, and communication. At the time of writing it remains the most comprehensive treatise on the subject.

The main conclusions of these reviews are summarised in Box 11.4.

BOX 11.4 MAIN CONCLUSIONS OF RECENT REVIEWS OF
ASSESSMENT OF PROFESSIONALISM IN MEDICAL EDUCATION[1-3,9-11]

- There is no single instrument for measuring 'professionalism.'
- Assessment of some elements of professionalism should take place over time.
- There is a need for 'triangulation', using more than one approach, method or instrument.
- Assessment should be carried out in as authentic a setting as possible (i.e. the workplace).
- Reliability can be improved by increasing the number of observations and observers.
- Judgements should be based on specific observations rather than relying upon recall.
- Assessment methods must be fair and transparent.
- There should be 'symmetry' within the 'system' (i.e. the same methods should be used at all levels).
- Both quantitative and qualitative methods should be developed.
- Lapses in professional behaviour and value conflicts, and the reasoning behind their resolution, should be assessed.

WORKPLACE-BASED ASSESSMENT

One of the most significant recent trends in healthcare education has been towards carrying out more assessment in the workplace. Here the focus is on how knowledge and skills are applied in everyday practice as opposed to how they are demonstrated under test or simulated conditions. An important underlying concept is that how someone behaves in real life (their so-called 'performance') is not predicted by how they behave under test conditions (their so-called 'competence') (*see* Box 11.3). This applies to all areas of professional practice, including demonstration of the attitudes that underpin professional practice. Miller, an American psychologist, proposed a framework for assessing clinical competence and performance, known as 'Miller's pyramid', with a hierarchy of levels or domains (*see* Figure 11.1).[12]

The lowest level focuses on what a person knows, and the highest level focuses on what a person does in practice. Ideally, assessment of professionalism should focus on the latter.

When thinking of appropriate methods for workplace-based assessment in clinical practice, several elements need to be considered:[13,14]

➤ the basis on which judgements are to be made (e.g. whether to look at the processes or at the outcomes of care)

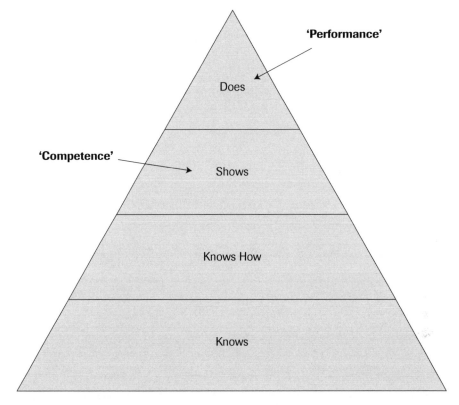

FIGURE 11.1 Miller's pyramid.[12]

➤ the data which inform the judgements (e.g. clinical records, performance data, observation of practice, etc.)
➤ the grounds for making the judgements (i.e. whether they are based on observation of single episodes, or on routine performance)
➤ the nature of those judgements (i.e. based on the quality or 'fitness for purpose' of observed performance, *or* simply whether something, such as a particular behaviour, was demonstrated or not).

Although ideally one might wish to evaluate patient outcomes, there are significant problems in doing this, given the complexity of healthcare and the increasingly team-based approach to its delivery. Few outcomes can be directly attributed to the actions of an individual professional, and thus team-based assessment of professionalism is a challenge for the future. Looking at *process* is easier because it is usually less dependent on what others do or on factors such as the patient's underlying health status. However, one of the main disadvantages is that it may only indicate that something has been done, and not how well it was done. Another consideration is how many encounters need to be observed in order to make valid and reliable judgements. The particular psychometric properties of the individual assessment instrument will guide practice, bearing in mind that the number required may vary according to its purpose – for example, whether it is to be used to identify unsatisfactory practice, or to grade and rank individuals. We would argue that assessment should be used for identifying good or unsatisfactory performance rather than for grading and ranking, but not all educators agree with this view.

Another issue is whether a checklist of behaviours or global ratings, with or without 'anchor statements', should be used (*see* Box 11.5). Although research has shown relatively little difference between them in terms of reliability, strictly speaking only experts should use global rating scales, and reliability is increased by using anchor statements and, of course, by training the assessors.

BOX 11.5 EXAMPLES OF GLOBAL RATING SCALE AND CHECKLIST

Global rating scale (with anchor statements)

Exemplary	*Satisfactory*	*Unsatisfactory*
Highly effective team member. Very good working relationships with other team members. Respectful of others' roles. Makes full and appropriate contributions. Excellent communication within the team	Generally effective team member with good working relationships. Respectful of others' roles, and contributes appropriately. Good communication within the team	Not an effective team member. Relationships with colleagues not always good. Does not show respect for others' roles

Checklist

Functions as highly effective team member	Exemplary – Satisfactory – Unsatisfactory
Has good working relationships	Exemplary – Satisfactory – Unsatisfactory
Shows respect for others' roles	Exemplary – Satisfactory – Unsatisfactory
Makes full and appropriate contributions	Exemplary – Satisfactory – Unsatisfactory
Demonstrates excellent communication	Exemplary – Satisfactory – Unsatisfactory

Several assessment instruments for use in the workplace have been developed in North America and the UK over the last few years, including the mini-CEX (mini-clinical evaluation exercise), DOPS (direct observation of procedural skills) and CBD (case-based discussion),[14] all of which are in common use in both undergraduate and postgraduate medical settings and, pertinently, all of which include 'professionalism' as one of the items for assessment.

John Norcini, a world authority on clinical assessment, has written about some of the challenges facing workplace-based assessment, including the effect of the relationship between the assessor and the assessed on the judgements made, how high the stakes of the assessment are (perhaps unsurprisingly, awarded grades tend to be higher in high-stakes situations!), and the feasibility of undertaking such assessment in the context of busy clinical practice.[14] One of the main challenges is concerned with reliability. This is affected by three main factors – the number of encounters observed, the number of observers, and the aspects of performance that are being observed. In general, the more encounters and observers there are the better, as the number of different areas of practice assessed has much less influence on reliability. Training assessors is also important.

REFLECTION AND SELF-ASSESSMENT

One of the key attributes of professionals is that they should be reflective (*see* Chapter 1). Indeed 'reflection' and 'the reflective practitioner' lie at the heart of most discussions about professionalism. Reflection is a crucial part of learning at all stages in the continuum of lifelong learning, enabling the individual to create meaning out of experience, to link theory to practice, and to identify further learning needs. Being able to explore their reflections should give learners insight into attitudes and perspectives on their role, what they have learned from a particular situation and what still needs to be learned. Reflection may also reveal their reasoning with regard to challenging professional dilemmas.[3] There are many theoretical approaches to and models of reflection, but they all share a number of principles. Reflection consists of a series of levels, ranging from superficial, descriptive levels to deep, analytical levels, and the deeper levels are regarded as harder to attain but have greater potential for learning.[15] There is also an obvious and dynamic relationship between reflection and the ability to assess one's own behaviour and practice accurately. Indeed one of the assumptions underlying the self-regulation historically enjoyed by the medical profession is that the competent professional is a self-directed learner, committed to lifelong learning (*see also* Chapter 7). Self-assessment (defined as 'a personal evaluation of one's professional attributes and abilities against perceived norms'[16]) is fundamental to the concept of self-directed learning.[15,17] Indeed it is highlighted as an important dimension of professionalism by healthcare regulating bodies such as the General Medical Council[18] and CanMEDS,[19] and it is a central plank of most systems of appraisal.[20]

Unfortunately, current evidence for self-assessment as an accurate and reliable process is not good. Indeed the very concept of the 'adult learner' has been challenged on these grounds.[21] Research in a wide range of subject areas, including medicine, has consistently shown that correlations between people's self-assessment and external measures are generally poor. The accuracy of global self-assessments over an extended period is particularly low, compounded by problems of recall.[22]

However, methodological problems in the research on self-assessment have been highlighted, and some of the underlying assumptions have been challenged.[22] Most of the studies look at the correlations between the subject's self-assessment and an external measure, usually an 'expert' evaluation. This assumes that experts are consistent in their judgements, yet there is evidence of inconsistency, especially when they are making judgements over time – experts are more likely to agree when observing short, structured tasks. A recent systematic review[16] concluded that there is evidence that the accuracy of self-assessment can be improved by feedback, especially verbal feedback or use of video review, and by providing explicit criteria for the process. There is also evidence to support the received wisdom that the least competent are the least able to self-assess accurately, often overestimating their capabilities, and the most competent may *under*estimate their own performance.

In the next section we discuss several approaches that are currently being used to assess aspects of professionalism, namely portfolios, assessment by peers, and assessment of communication.

PORTFOLIO-BASED ASSESSMENT

Portfolios originated in areas such as art and architecture. They have been used outside medicine for many years, and at all levels from elementary to higher education, including vocational and professional programmes, for a variety of purposes – both formative and summative. The use of portfolios has been gaining ground in medicine in the past decade, despite considerable resistance and scepticism, and is now embedded at various stages in the continuum of medical education. A portfolio-based approach is congruent with the nature of professional practice and how professionals learn. However, the most contentious area remains the role of portfolios in assessment (as opposed to enhancement of learning and professional development). For example, there is concern about their reliability in high-stakes situations.[23]

What is a portfolio?

The portfolio, defined as a collection of material compiled over a period of time and brought together for a specific purpose,[24] is not an assessment method as such but more a format for organising assessment. In theory, a portfolio can include a wide range of material – by definition anything that provides appropriate evidence of whatever is being assessed, including learning plans, lists of procedures and tasks undertaken, case reports, evaluations of performance and behaviour by self, peers, supervisors, other members of a team or patients, videotapes of interactions with patients, results of audits or research, published work, testimonials, critical incidents, and (some would argue crucially) reflective writing (e.g. evaluating the evidence and reflecting on personal growth and development). The content will obviously be defined by the intended purpose of the portfolio and, in the words of one author, 'Evidence in portfolios is limited only by the degree of the designer's creativity.'[25] Arguments have been made in favour of portfolios being flexible enough to allow people to include self-selected material. Another way of looking at a portfolio is that it is a learning plan with evidence – the collected material is the evidence that stated objectives have been achieved.[26] However, for both practical and technical reasons, a degree of standardisation of both structure and content is probably necessary, especially if the portfolio has any summative function (see below). Until recently portfolios tended to be paper based, although there seems to be an inexorable trend towards the development and use of electronic portfolios.

Why use a portfolio-based approach?

At least in theory, a portfolio-based approach creates a closer link between the processes of learning and assessment. With regard to assessment of professionalism, a portfolio approach attempts to assess complex areas such as attitudes, personal attributes and reflective ability, offering an alternative to the limitations of the traditional approaches to assessment in medicine (e.g. multiple-choice questions). In taking account of the context of personal and professional development, its highly personalised nature is acknowledged. Since a portfolio is usually completed over time, it takes account of the developmental nature of professionalism. The advantages of a portfolio-based approach that have been proposed by various authors are listed in Box 11.6.

BOX 11.6 ADVANTAGES OF A PORTFOLIO-BASED APPROACH TO ASSESSMENT[24-26]

- Can assess areas that have been found difficult to test conventionally.
- Encapsulates the principles of adult learning.
- Can incorporate a range of methods – both qualitative and quantitative.
- Assesses more authentic, workplace-based contexts.
- Promotes links between theory and practice.
- Stimulates use of reflective strategies.
- May be able to identify poor performance at an early stage.
- Promotes creativity.
- Can demonstrate progression and development (as opposed to simply providing a 'snapshot').
- Promotes development of strategies for lifelong learning.
- Provides a profile of learners' competencies and achievements.
- Enhances interactions between learners and teachers/supervisors.
- Takes account of individual learning styles and preferences.

BOX 11.7 DISADVANTAGES OF A PORTFOLIO-BASED APPROACH TO ASSESSMENT

- Concerns about reliability.
- Possibility of plagiarism and fabrication.
- Time constraints (for both the learner and the assessor).
- Cost.
- Negative attitudes towards the process.

However, there are a number of potential disadvantages to the use of port-folios, as outlined in Box 11.7. A major issue is their reliability, especially in the context of their use in 'high-stakes' settings, when decisions about progress, selection and/or qualification will be based on assessment results. To quote a recent commentary, 'the evidence backing the widespread introduction for high-stakes summative assessments is thin, to say the least, and many gaps are evident.'[23] However, there has been a move towards adopting a qualitative ap-proach in which validity is seen as the more relevant dimension, an important element of which is the trustworthiness of the data. This raises the need to demonstrate that the content is authentic, that there is sufficient evidence and that it is current among other factors.[27] With regard to its utility (see above), a portfolio-based approach carries a significant cost in terms of investment of time – for the learner to compile the evidence, for the assessor to appraise it, and for the necessary discussions about the material to take place. Ideally assessors also need training. This affects the acceptability of this approach.

Implementing portfolio-based assessment

Guidelines for implementing a portfolio-based approach have been described,[4,26,27] and include being clear about the purpose and content, providing clear instructions for use, ensuring that the criteria used for making judgements are transparent, and evaluating the process. There is little doubt that the use of portfolios in the assessment of professionalism will continue to develop.

COMMUNICATION

At the core of patient-centred professionalism is the interaction between the doctor and the patient, and this is an obvious and important focus for assessment of professionalism. Taking a broader view, effective communication is a key component in many other aspects of professional practice, including teamwork, as well as in the prevention of error.[28] Patient–doctor communication is an area in which there has been a huge amount of research and development, in parallel with the growth of teaching and training in communication. An evidence base is emerging that demonstrates the benefits of good communication.[29,30] Frameworks such as the Calgary–Cambridge approach break down the consultation into its constituent 'microskills', which in turn enables detailed assessment.[29] Routine assessment of communication is now embedded in medical training and professional development at both undergraduate and postgraduate levels, and is evolving all the time. However, it has been a long time coming. Until relatively recently, communication was not formally assessed at *any* level (indeed it was not formally taught either). It was assumed that appropriate communication techniques would be picked up by 'osmosis', and that demonstration of mastery of knowledge and technical skills was sufficient to guarantee clinical competence. Despite accumulating evidence to the contrary, it has only been in the last couple of decades that the profession has taken communication skills teaching and assessment seriously.[30-32]

There is a wide variety of approaches to assessment of communication, some of which will be discussed in the section below, but the reader is directed to more comprehensive reviews for further detail (e.g. Thistlethwaite J, Morris P. *The Patient-Doctor Consultation in Primary Care*. London: Royal College of General Practitioners; 2006).

The structured OSCE station, now widely used in healthcare education, commonly assesses communication at the level of specific microskills and behaviours. With regard to van der Vleuten's utility equation (*see* Box 11.2), OSCEs, depending on factors such as the total test time and the number and range of cases, are generally reliable, acceptable and can drive learning in more or less appropriate directions. However, since they are not holistic assessments because they (necessarily) abstract microskills from the 'bigger picture', their validity can be questionable, and of course they are highly resource-intensive. The OSCE can drive learning in a way that promotes a formulaic approach to consultation, with candidates 'going through the motions' without perhaps genuinely interacting with the patient (e.g. eliciting the patient's concerns but not responding to them). Furthermore, a checklist marking scheme may actually reward this kind of approach. This problem is compounded by the inevitable time constraints of an OSCE in which, typically, candidates only have a few minutes in which to perform a complex task, such as explaining treatment options, that in real life we would expect to take much longer (indeed we would admonish our learners if they took short cuts). Finally, OSCEs assess competence ('shows how'), not performance ('does') (*see* Box 11.3). Other challenges include achieving the right balance of communication and other skills both within individual stations and across the whole examination or teaching programme, and the fact that, since both competence and performance are content-specific, a large number of stations may be required to assess specific elements of communication in professionalism – for example, assessment of empathy, for which one study suggested 37 cases/ stations would be required![33]

In the UK, the Royal College of General Practitioners (RCGP) took the OSCE approach one stage further in their membership examination in which candidates could undertake a simulated surgery (or clinic) consisting of several cases involving simulated patients presenting with a wide variety of conditions. It was shown to be a valid and reliable tool for assessing a wide range of competencies.[34] Building on this, the RCGP has gone on to develop a new integrated clinical skills assessment for membership, in which consultation skills and other dimensions of professionalism are embedded.[35] Workplace-based assessments such as the mini-CEX referred to earlier also attempt to assess in a more holistic way, and usually include aspects of communication alongside technical skills.

There are several approaches to assessing communication in the workplace, including direct observation (assessor sitting in on real consultations), videotaping and evaluating consultations, and seeking the views of either real patients or incognito simulated patients (the 'mystery shopper').[36] These are briefly discussed below.

Direct observation is usually used for formative purposes. An advantage is that feedback can be given immediately. A disadvantage is that the presence of the observer will inevitably influence the behaviour of the person who is being observed, and thus any assessment is more likely to be of their competence than of their performance. Videotaping and analysis of consultations have been used for assessment purposes in general practice training for over 25 years (e.g. the exit summative assessment at the end of the vocational training programme in the UK). Methods and instruments have been developed to a high level of sophistication and have good psychometric properties. One example of such an instrument is the Leicester Assessment Package.[37,38] Real patients can be asked for feedback about a doctor's communication skills. Although they may not be able to judge technical issues reliably, only patients can say whether they felt valued, and whether the doctor gave them enough time, listened to their concerns, involved them in decisions about their care, and explained things effectively. Patients' views can be solicited either immediately after the consultation or some time later (e.g. by questionnaire or telephone interview). Indeed, all GPs in the UK are now contractually required to carry out regular surveys using one of several validated tools. The areas usually observed include provision of time, exploration of patients' needs, listening, explaining, giving information and sharing decisions. Interpersonal attributes include humaneness, caring, supporting and trust. One such measure is the General Practice Assessment Questionnaire (GPAQ).[39] This was developed from a research tool called the General Practice Assessment Survey (GPAS), itself based on an American instrument, the Primary Care Assessment Survey. For the GP contract, the original GPAS questionnaire was modified and shortened and is available in two versions, one designed to be sent by post and one designed to be given to patients after consultations in the surgery. A version for use by nurses has also been developed. Based on extensive evaluation, it is recommended that questionnaires from around 50 patients per GP (fewer for larger practices) will be enough to show up important differences between doctors or practices.[39]

The role of incognito (covert) simulated patients in assessing doctors' performance is controversial. Simulated or standardised patients have been shown to be able to judge consistently many aspects of students' or doctors' competence in exams.[40] However, a recent systematic review of the literature on incognito standardised patients (ISPs) concluded that the added value of this approach was still uncertain, and that there were also unanswered questions about consistency and accuracy. The authors did not think that the use of ISPs would be 'the final solution' to the challenge of assessing performance.[41] There are also ethical issues relating to consent of the participating doctors, as well as questions about how the results are fed back. Nonetheless, the authors felt that it was an exciting area and that further research was necessary.

ASSESSMENT BY PEERS

The idea of being judged by one's peers when going about one's daily business has, in theory, much to offer. Peers have a unique perspective, because we let our guard down in their company (compared with when we are under direct observation), and they can provide insight into behaviours that are distinctly different from those based on information from other sources. Peer assessment is now found in virtually all areas of professional practice. As mentioned previously, reliability is mainly influenced by the number of observations, the number of observers and the number of 'things' being observed. The context and setting are obviously also important influences, as are relationships and whether or not the assessment is summative and 'high stakes.'

Evans and colleagues undertook a systematic review of the literature on peer assessment in medicine.[42] Three rating scales were identified, all of which were developed in North America and all of which were intended for formative purposes. Unfortunately, there was little data on the respective instruments' development and theoretical basis, and problems were identified with their psychometric properties – for example, questions about reliability (which was modest) and aspects of validity. Based on their review, the authors concluded that 'peer assessment methods should be used with caution.'[42] However, other authors have demonstrated that peer assessment *can* be a reasonable measure of interpersonal and communication skills, relationships with colleagues and patients, and humanity.[2] The approach is acceptable to learners so long as certain criteria are met, including a supportive environment, complete anonymity and prompt feedback. The process must focus on both the positives and negatives, and should be used formatively, rewarding exemplary behaviour as well as identifying lapses in professional behaviour.[43]

Notwithstanding these concerns, multi-source feedback (MSF) is increasing in popularity in medicine, having been used for many years in industry. There is also a growing evidence base to support its use.[44,45] MSF involves collecting and collating feedback, usually via a questionnaire, from a group of colleagues and possibly patients. It has the potential to influence practice through generation of structured feedback which identifies both a person's strengths and areas for development. Two MSF tools in common usage in the UK are the Sheffield Peer Review Assessment Tool (SPRAT), and a modified version known as the miniPAT which was developed specifically for the Foundation Programme for doctors (interns).[46,47] The former consists of 24 questions with

BOX 11.8 THE MINIPAT MULTI-SOURCE FEEDBACK INSTRUMENT

Please refer to curriculum at www.mmc.nhs.uk for details of expected competencies for F1 and F2

mini-PAT (Peer Assessment Tool) - F2 Version

Please complete the questions using a cross: ☒   Please use black ink and CAPITAL LETTERS

Doctor's   Surname

Forename

GMC Number:

How do you rate this Doctor in their:	Below expectations for F2 completion	Borderline for F2 completion	Meets expectations for F2 completion		Above expectations for F2 completion		U/C*
	1	2	3	4	5	6	
Good Clinical Care							
1 Ability to diagnose patient problems	☐	☐	☐	☐	☐	☐	☐
2 Ability to formulate appropriate management plans	☐	☐	☐	☐	☐	☐	☐
3 Awareness of their own limitations	☐	☐	☐	☐	☐	☐	☐
4 Ability to respond to psychosocial aspects of illness	☐	☐	☐	☐	☐	☐	☐
5 Appropriate utilisation of resources e.g. ordering investigations	☐	☐	☐	☐	☐	☐	☐
Maintaining good medical practice							
6 Ability to manage time effectively / prioritise	☐	☐	☐	☐	☐	☐	☐
7 Technical skills (appropriate to current practice)	☐	☐	☐	☐	☐	☐	☐
Teaching and Training, Appraising and Assessing							
8 Willingness and effectiveness when teaching/training colleagues	☐	☐	☐	☐	☐	☐	☐
Relationship with Patients							
9 Communication with patients	☐	☐	☐	☐	☐	☐	☐
10 Communication with carers and/or family	☐	☐	☐	☐	☐	☐	☐
11 Respect for patients and their right to confidentiality	☐	☐	☐	☐	☐	☐	☐
Working with colleagues							
12 Verbal communication with colleagues	☐	☐	☐	☐	☐	☐	☐
13 Written communication with colleagues	☐	☐	☐	☐	☐	☐	☐
14 Ability to recognise and value the contribution of others	☐	☐	☐	☐	☐	☐	☐
15 Accessibility/Reliability	☐	☐	☐	☐	☐	☐	☐
16 Overall, how do you rate this doctor compared to a doctor ready to complete F2 training?	☐	☐	☐	☐	☐	☐	☐

Do you have any concerns about this doctor's probity or health?   ☐ Yes   ☐ No
If yes please state your concerns:

*U/C Please mark this if you have not observed the behaviour and therefore feel unable to comment.   2500288218

Anything especially good?

Please describe any behaviour that has raised concerns or should be a particular focus for development:

Please continue your comments on a separate sheet if required

Your Gender:	☐ Male	☐ Female

Your ethnic group:

☐ British   ☐ Bangladeshi

☐ Irish   ☐ Other Asian Background

☐ Other White Background   ☐ White and Black Caribbean

☐ Caribbean   ☐ White and Black African

☐ African   ☐ White and Asian

☐ Any other Black background   ☐ Any other mixed background

☐ Indian   ☐ Chinese

☐ Pakistani   ☐ Any other ethnic group

Which environment have you primarily observed the doctor in?
(Please choose one answer only)

☐ Inpatients   ☐ Intensive Care

☐ Outpatients   ☐ Theatre

☐ Both In and Out-patients   ☐ General Practice

☐ A&E/Admissions   ☐ Other (Please specify)

☐ Community Speciality

☐ Laboratory/Research

Your position:

☐ Consultant   ☐ SASG   ☐ SpR   ☐ Foundation/PRHO

☐ Nurse   ☐ SHO   ☐ Allied Health Professional

☐ GP

☐ Other (Please specify)

If you are a Nurse or AHP how long have you been qualified?: ☐☐ years

Length of working relationship: ☐☐ months

What training have you had in the use of this assessment tool?: ☐ Face-to-Face   ☐ Have Read Guidelines   ☐ Web/CD rom

How long has it taken you to complete this form (in minutes)?: ☐☐

Your Signature: _____ Date: ☐☐ / ☐☐ / ☐☐

Your Surname: ☐☐☐☐☐☐☐☐☐☐☐☐☐☐☐☐☐☐☐☐☐☐☐

Your GMC Number: (Doctors only) ☐☐☐☐☐☐☐

Acknowledgements: mini-PAT is derived from SPRAT (Sheffield Peer Review Assessment Tool)

9787288212

a 6-point rating scale, a global rating and space for free-text comments, and the latter consists of 15 questions (*see* Box 11.8). The person is also asked to nominate eight 'peers' to approach for feedback.

Psychometric testing and evaluation have shown in fact that as few as four raters may be sufficient to make a confident judgement as to whether someone is having problems. For 'borderline' doctors, more raters may be needed. Surprisingly, the use of self-nominated raters – which is the norm – does not appear to affect ratings. The person who is being assessed receives their own ratings compared with the mean ratings by their peer group. The effectiveness and utility of the instrument depend crucially on the quality of the feedback, which begs the need for faculty development in this area.

RESPONDING TO LAPSES IN PROFESSIONALISM

One further challenge is how to and who should respond when assessment identifies someone whose 'professionalism' is in question. Minor lapses may simply be noted in the learner's file. Persistent unacceptable behaviours may trigger a discussion with a senior colleague (e.g. an educational supervisor), associated with a warning (analogous to football's Yellow Card). More serious and/or chronic lapses will need to invoke some kind of 'fitness to practise' appraisal. It is our experience, at both undergraduate and postgraduate levels, that there is often both a failure to detect and a reluctance to respond to minor lapses. One author referred to 'the blind eye and conspiracy of silence', and went on to state that 'We are inclined to remain silent about exemplary behaviour and excuse, rationalize or lament lapses in professionalism.'[48] There are many possible reasons for this (*see* Box 11.9).

In line with developments in the postgraduate arena (e.g. the GMC's procedures for dealing with poorly performing doctors[49]), medical schools have been exhorted to develop robust 'fitness to practise' procedures. The GMC put the issue into the broader context of the duties of a doctor when it issued guidance to medical schools about how to deal with medical students' behaviour and fitness to practise.[50]

How to manage poor performance, particularly in practising doctors, is a major challenge. Whereas assessment systems are generally well developed, it has been observed that systems for remediation (defined as an intervention, or suite of interventions, required in response to assessment against threshold standards of performance.'[51]) are not so, at least in North America and the UK, and that they lack consistency of approach and methods.[51,52] A number of key principles underpin success in developing and managing a system for remediation, including ensuring that interventions are customised, that subjects are engaged and thus motivated to participate, and that such systems have institutional support while those professionals involved in the process are able to maintain an independent stance (to enable a trusting relationship to develop).[51] Reasons for underperformance are complex, dynamic and idiosyncratic. Therefore any system for remediation needs to interface with a wide range of agencies, such as occupational health and physical and mental health services (mental health problems and substance misuse commonly underpin poor performance). Approaches that have been explored include cognitive behavioural therapy and motivational interviewing.[51]

BOX 11.9 REASONS WHY LAPSES IN PROFESSIONALISM MIGHT GO UNNOTICED

- Appropriate tools are not available, and there is not a system for responding.
- Increased numbers of learners mean that there is limited time for meaningful interaction and observation.
- 'Whistleblowing' is frowned upon within the profession.
- Concerns about the subjectivity of the instrument and consequent judgements.
- Concerns about adversely influencing progression (whether academic or career).
- Perceived lack of skills to tackle the issue.
- The probability of impairing working relationships.
- Concern about comeback, complaints or litigation.

FINAL THOUGHTS

Medical educators and their institutions have made a big investment in developing and evaluating approaches to measuring professionalism, with promising results in a wide range of areas. Many of these have been discussed in this chapter, albeit superficially on account of the scale of the enterprise. However, this area also has a high media profile, invariably as a result of blatant failures of self-regulation on the part of the medical profession, so the public and politicians are to a certain extent breathing down the medical profession's neck. Nonetheless, we need to keep returning to the underlying concepts to remind ourselves about the nature of the beast, and not only to reflect on the reasons why we need to measure professionalism (we are now fairly confident, for example, that there is evidence that negative behaviour as a student is correlated with less desirable behaviours later in an individual's career[52-54]), but also to remind ourselves of the challenges.

Fred Hafferty from Minnesota will be given the last word on assessment of professionalism. In a very thoughtful commentary in Stern's definitive text,[2] he raises a number of concerns. He argues that we must guard against reducing professionalism to what he calls 'a static thing' independent of its context, and observes that by reducing it to a set of observable behaviours for the purposes of teaching and assessment we demean it and are likely to induce a kind of 'surface professionalism', and may thus miss important elements. He reminds us that professionalism is developmental and changing, that it is actually highly context-specific, and he contends that attainment of the status of 'professional' should be problematic, not automatic, and that maintenance of that status should be treated as contingent, not complementary. Finally, he discusses a range of issues related to assessment of professionalism, including the use of language and the importance of context. He concludes by lamenting the rise of managed care and commercialisation in medicine, alongside the often questionable probity and the avarice of clinicians (e.g. in relation to the pharmaceutical industry), which demonstrates one set of values – those that underpin 'professionalism' in its broadest sense. Medical educators cannot accomplish what needs to be done on their own. Change can only come about as a result of a cultural shift at institutional level: 'If organized medicine truly desires professionalism . . . then organized medicine is going to have to say "there's a new sheriff in town" – and mean it.'[2]

REFERENCES

1 Lynch DC, Surdyk PM, Esier AR. Assessing professionalism: a review of the literature. *Med Teach.* 2004; **26**: 366–73.

2 Stern DT, editor. *Measuring Medical Professionalism*. Oxford: Oxford University Press; 2006.

3 Ginsburg S, Regehr G, Hatala R *et al.* Context, conflict and resolution: a new conceptual framework for evaluating professionalism. *Acad Med.* 2000; **75**: S6–11.

4 Harden RM, Lilley PM. Best evidence medical education: the simple truth. *Med Teach.* 2000; **22**: 117–19.

5 Van der Vleuten CPM. The assessment of professional competence: developments, research and practical implications. *Adv Health Sci Educ.* 1996; **1**: 41–67.

6 Crossley J, Davies H, Humphris G *et al.* Generalisability: a key to unlock professional assessment. *Med Educ.* 2002; **36**: 972–8.

7 Schurwith L. Professional development in undergraduate medical curricula from an assessment point of view. *Med Educ.* 2002; **36**: 312–13.

8 Norcini J. The death of the long case? *BMJ.* 2002; **324**: 408–9.

9 Arnold L. Assessing professional behaviour: yesterday, today, and tomorrow. *Acad Med.* 2002; **77**: 502–15.

10 Veloski JJ, Fields SK, Boex JR *et al.* Measuring professionalism: a review of studies with instruments reported in the literature between 1982 and 2002. *Acad Med.* 2005; **80:** 366–70.

11 Epstein RE, Hundert EM. Defining and assessing professional competence. *JAMA.* 2002; **287:** 226–35.

12 Miller GE. The assessment of clinical skills/competence/performance. *Acad Med.* 1990; **65 (Suppl. 9):** S63–7.

13 Norcini JJ. ABC of learning and teaching in medicine. Work-based assessment. *BMJ.* 2003; **326:** 753–5.

14 Norcini JJ. *Workplace-Based Assessment in Clinical Training.* Edinburgh: Association for the Study of Medical Education; 2007.

15 Kaufmann DM, Mann KV. *Teaching and Learning in Medical Education: how theory can inform practice.* Edinburgh: Association for the Study of Medical Education; 2007.

16 McKinstry B *et al.* BEME systematic review: the effectiveness of self-assessment on the identification of learner needs, learner activity and impact on clinical practice; www.bemecollaboration.org/beme/files/BEME%20Guide%20No%2010/ BEMEFinalReportSA240108.pdf (accessed April 2008).

17 Spencer JA, Jordan RK. Learner-centred approaches in medical education. *BMJ.* 1999; **318:** 1280–83.

18 General Medical Council. *Good Medical Practice.* London: General Medical Council; 2006.

19 http://rcpsc.medical.org/canmeds/index.php (accessed September 2007).

20 www.dh.gov.uk/en/Publicationsandstatistics/Publications/PublicationsPolicyAnd Guidance/DH_4006979 (accessed September 2007).

21 Norman G. The adult learner: a mythical species? *Acad Med.* 1999; **74:** 886–9.

22 Ward M, Gruppen L, Regehr G. Measuring self-assessment: current state of the art. *Adv Health Sci Educ.* 2002; **7:** 63–80.

23 Roberts C, Newble D, O'Rourke AJ. Portfolio-based assessments in medical education: are they valid and reliable for summative purposes? *Med Educ.* 2002; **36:** 899–900.

24 Challis M. Portfolio-based learning and assessment in medical education. *Med Teach.* 1999; **21:** 370–86.

25 Friedman Ben-David M, Davis MH, Harden RM *et al.* Portfolios as a method of student assessment. *Med Teach.* 2001; **23:** 535–51.

26 Thistlethwaite JE. How to keep a portfolio. *Clin Teach.* 2006; **3:** 118–23.

27 Pitts J. *Portfolios, Personal Development and Reflective Practice.* Edinburgh: Association for the Study of Medical Education; 2007.

28 Hays R, Davies HA, Beard JD *et al.* Selecting performance assessment methods for experienced physicians. *Med Educ.* 2002; **36:** 910–17.

29 Silverman J, Kurtz S, Draper J. *Skills for Communicating with Patients.* 2nd ed. Oxford: Radcliffe Publishing; 2005.

30 Makoul G, Curry RH. The value of assessing and addressing communication skills. *JAMA.* 2007; **298:** 1057–9.

31 Makoul G, Schofield T. Communication teaching and assessment in medical education: an international consensus statement. *Patient Educ Counsel.* 1999; **37:** 191–5.

32 Simpson M, Buckman R, Stewart M *et al.* Doctor–patient communication: the Toronto Consensus Statement. *BMJ.* 1991; **303:** 1385–7.

33 Colliver JA, Willis MS, Robbs RS *et al.* Assessment of empathy in a standardized patient examination. *Teach Learn Med.* 1998; **10:** 8–11.

34 Burrows PJ, Bingham L. The simulated surgery – an alternative to videotape submission for the consulting skills component of the MRCGP examination: the first year's experience. *Br J Gen Pract.* 1999; **49:** 269–72.

35 Wass V. A guide to the new MRCGP exam. *BMJ Career Focus.* 2005; **331:** 158–9.

36 Thistlethwaite J, Morris P. Assessment of communication/consultation skills and competence. In: Thistlethwaite J, Morris P. *The Patient–Doctor Consultation in Primary Care.* London: Royal College of General Practitioners; 2006.

37 Fraser RC, McKinley RK, Mulholland H. Consultation competence in general practice: establishing the face validity of prioritized criteria of the Leicester assessment package. *Br J Gen Pract.* 1994; **44:** 109–13.

38 Fraser RC, McKinley RK, Mulholland H. Consultation competence in general practice: testing the reliability of the Leicester assessment package. *Br J Gen Pract.* 1994; **44:** 293–6.

39 www.gpaq.info (accessed February 2007).

40 Thistlethwaite J, Ridgway G. *Making it Real: a practical guide to experiential learning of communication skills.* Oxford: Radcliffe Publishing; 2006.

41 Rethans J-J, Gorter S, Bokken L *et al.* Unannounced standardised patients in real practice: a systematic literature review. *Med Educ.* 2007; **41:** 537–49.

42 Evans R, Elwyn G, Edwards A. Review of instruments for peer assessment of physicians. *BMJ.* 2004; **328:** 1240–43.

43 Arnold L, Shue CK, Kalishman S *et al.* Can there be a single system for peer assessment of professionalism among medical students? A multi-institutional study. *Acad Med.* 2007; **82:** 578–86.

44 Lockyer J. Multisource feedback in the assessment of physician competencies. *J Contin Educ Health Prof.* 2003; **23:** 4–12.

45 Norcini J. Peer assessment of competence. *Med Educ.* 2003; **37:** 539–43.

46 Davies H, Archer J. Multi-source feedback: development and practical aspects. *Clin Teach.* 2005; **2:** 77–81.

47 www.google.co.uk/search?hl=en&q=+MMC+Foundation&btnG=Search&meta= (accessed February 2008).

48 Arnold L. Responding to the professionalism of learners and faculty in orthopaedic surgery. *Clin Orthop Relat Res.* 2006; **449:** 205–13.

49 www.gmc-uk.org/concerns/index.asp (accessed February 2008).

50 www.gmc-uk.org/education/documents/Medical_students_Professional_behaviour_and_ftp.pdf (accessed February 2008).

51 Cohen D, Rhydderch M, Cooper I. *Managing Remediation.* Edinburgh: Association for the Study of Medical Education; 2007.

52 Papadakis MA, Hodgson CS, Teherani A *et al.* Unprofessional behaviour in medical school is associated with subsequent disciplinary action by a state medical board. *Acad Med.* 2004; **79:** 244–9.

53 Papadakis MA, Teherani A, Banach MA *et al.* Disciplinary action by medical boards and prior behaviour in medical school. *NEJM.* 2005; **353:** 2673–82.

54 Teherani A, Hodgson CS, Banach M *et al.* Domains of unprofessional behaviour during medical school associated with future disciplinary action by a state medical board. *Acad Med.* 2005; **80 (Suppl. 10):** S17–20.

CHAPTER 12

Professionalism and social justice: the next step?

This chapter explores:
- the concept of social justice
- the widening healthcare gap
- further thoughts on altruism
- patients' needs
- rationing of healthcare
- the responsibility of health professionals.

> Health is a state of complete physical, mental and social well-being and not merely the absence of disease or infirmity. The enjoyment of the highest attainable standard of health is one of the fundamental rights of every human being without distinctions of race, political belief, economic or social condition.
>
> *World Health Organization, 1946*[1]

This chapter considers some of the themes discussed in earlier chapters from a different perspective – that of social justice. The international Medical Professionalism Project (founded in 1999 by the European Federation of Internal Medicine, the American College of Physicians and the American Board of Internal Medicine) acknowledges the primacy of patient welfare and social justice, including the fair distribution of healthcare resources, as attributes of professionalism.[2] The concept of social justice brings together several of the themes of professionalism, namely those of ethics and law, altruism and, obliquely, self-care. The extent to which health professionals should become involved in areas that appear to be the province of politicians and government is certainly open to debate. Although we are sure that most readers would agree that health professionals should provide the best healthcare possible within their own chosen field of expertise, how far should they go to champion the cause of their country's citizens and in particular those citizens who are not strictly their own patients? We would also ask the following question. Is there any onus on health professionals to campaign for fair health provision in the poorer nations of the world?

The definition of and ethical issues relating to rights were explored in Chapter 3. We briefly touched on rationing in Chapter 9, when discussing clinical governance and clinical audit. We mentioned that Richard Smith, previous editor of the *British Medical Journal*, criticised the National Institute for Health and Clinical Excellence (NICE) as being primarily concerned with rationing healthcare.[3] Although many doctors and allied health professionals may not see that one of their roles is fighting against national and international inequity in healthcare access and provision, we would argue that professionals should be able to debate rationing decisions, consider their ethical anteced-ents, and be champions of a fair distribution of resources.

This may be at a very local level, such as lobbying for healthcare facilities to remain open or to be upgraded, or on a larger stage, such as being involved in the fight for social justice on a national or world scale. Simply defined, social justice is about the management and delivery of healthcare in a fair and just way to all, regardless of means, gender or race. However, philosophically and practically there is a lot more to it than can be conveyed in one sentence (*see* Box 12.1).

BOX 12.1 SOME DEFINITIONS

Just: Based on behaving according to what is morally right and fair.

Justice: Just behaviour or treatment – the quality of being fair and reasonable.[4]

Social justice: Giving people a fair share or a choice based on their human rights as defined by the 1948 United Nations Universal Declaration of Human Rights.[5]

SOCIAL JUSTICE

It is impossible for all human beings to be equally healthy. Genetic conditions, chronic disease and accidents mitigate against this at the present time. However, a condition of equity is that patients in similar circumstances are treated in similar ways. Is it possible to treat all people equally within a health service? It certainly does not seem possible within most societies. The research literature shows that the richer one is, the longer and healthier one's life is. The Black Report demonstrated this a quarter of a century ago.[6] This is not just a question of access to a doctor or other health professional, the number of doctors being trained, the distance to secondary care facilities or the availability of state-of-the-art medical equipment. The main determinants of health are gender, culture, genetic make-up and social determinants, such as education, social organisation, income, diet and the environment.[7] Of course some of these are not amenable to manipulation. However, the social determinants of health affect morbidity and mortality across the spectrum of disease (both acute and chronic), and these social determinants are largely related to wealth. Quality of and access to education depend on government policies. How may health professionals influence this? The American philosopher Norman Daniels has proposed four conditions which, once achieved, will help to eliminate injustices in health outcomes (*see* Box 12.2).[8]

BOX 12.2 CONDITIONS NEEDED FOR SOCIAL JUSTICE

- Equal liberties.
- Robustly equal opportunities.
- Fair distribution of resources.
- Support for people's self-respect.

A country's prosperity is related to health as measured by its life expectancy – citizens of the rich nations of the world tend to live longer. However, wealth is not the only factor involved, as mentioned above. For example, people in Costa Rica live on average 2 years longer than people in the USA, although of course the Gross National Product of the USA far exceeds that of Costa Rica.[8] One of the main reasons for this discrepancy is the distribution of wealth within a country. 'Differences in health outcomes among developed nations cannot be explained simply by the absolute deprivation associated with low economic development – lack of access to the basic material conditions necessary for health, such as clean water, adequate nutrition and housing, and general sanitary living conditions. The degree of relative deprivation within a society also matters.'[8] The gap between rich and poor in most countries is growing. The socio-economic gradient runs parallel to life expectancy. In other words, inequality affects health status. The most egalitarian societies of the world tend to have the best health.[9]

AN EXAMPLE FROM AUSTRALIA

The histories of the indigenous nations of the world, those living in countries colonised or invaded (depending on your point of view) by mainly European powers, are good examples of how social and cultural inequities affect health-care and heath status. Consider the statistics shown in Box 12.3 relating to the Aboriginal and Torres Strait Islanders (the indigenous people) of Australia.

BOX 12.3 INDIGENOUS HEALTHCARE STATISTICS[10]

- At best, the life expectancy for Aborigines at birth is 12–15 years shorter than that of other Australians, and at worst the difference is 20 years.
- Male Aborigines expect to live on average to 56 years of age, and females to 62.7 years.
- The infant mortality rate of 13.6 per 1000 live births is three times higher than the non-indigenous rate.
- The prevalence of type 2 diabetes is 10–30%, which is two to four times higher than the non-indigenous rate.
- Renal failure is endemic.
- The prevalence of ischaemic heart disease and stroke is about three times higher than the non-indigenous rate.
- A higher proportion of Aboriginal people are non-drinkers compared with non-Aboriginal Australians, but of those Aboriginal people who do drink alcohol, a higher proportion drink at levels hazardous to health.
- The unemployment rate at 23% is three times higher than the national average.
- Violence against women is a major problem. Remote Indigenous women are 19 times more likely to be admitted to hospital due to assault and 10 times more likely to die from assault than other Australian women.

There are complex reasons for such figures, including loss of cultural identity, dispossession of land, changing diet and exercise patterns, alienation and racial prejudice, to name just a few. Health professionals working within Australia need to be aware of the health and social needs of these people, and in order to understand these needs they have to have an awareness of the history and life stories of the indigenous community. Cultural safety training is an important part of a health professional's development, but is not mandatory in many sectors.

Even if health professionals do not feel that it is part of their remit to try to bring about political change with regard to examples of social inequity, it is their professional duty to be equipped to communicate and understand the perspective of indigenous people within the countries within which they practise. Similarly, it is their duty to explore the perspective of immigrants to their country, as discussed in Chapter 6.

DOCTORS' PLACE IN SOCIETY

In the richest nations of the world, doctors are usually ranked within the higher earners, and are seen to be so by the patients for whom they care. Consider the stereotypical scenario in Box 12.4. What does this say about social justice, the social position of doctors and their relationship to their patients?

BOX 12.4 DR S AND SALLY M

Dr S has been qualified for 25 years. She was the first person from her working-class family to go to medical school. She received almost a full student grant from the government, and did not have to pay any university fees. After five years of hard work she graduated with only a small overdraft. Now she is a successful GP and works in a semi-rural practice in the North of England. Her annual remuneration is such that she is in the top income tax bracket of 40%. The practice population includes wealthy professionals, farmers, manual labourers and a fair number of unemployed patients. Her last patient of the morning is Sally M, a 19-year-old single mother of two children. Sally rang for a home visit, but was told to come down as an extra at the end of surgery. Sally is 15 minutes late, and Dr S had been just about to leave the building. Sally struggles in with 3-year-old toddler Ben and 6-month-old baby Darren, who is crying inconsolably. She has had to walk two miles from her housing estate because the bus was late. In the past Dr S has advised Sally to give up smoking and lose weight. She is unhappy that Sally is not breastfeeding Darren. She tells Sally it is no wonder that Darren is ill again. Dr S repeats her previous advice about Ben's diet. He is eating too much junk food. Dr S is frustrated that Sally does not appear to be listening to her and makes no effort to change her lifestyle. Sally tells the doctor that she has been hoping to go to college but her grandmother, who usually babysits, is becoming more immobile due to her arthritis. Mrs M has been on the waiting list for a hip replacement for over 8 months. However, Dr S forgets about Sally as she gets ready for a weekend off. First she drives in her new Audi to the nearby private hospital to see her mother, who has just had a knee replacement. The specialist was able to fit her in a week after seeing her in the clinic. Then she goes home. Her daughter, who is studying at a private school in the local town, has an interview for medical school the following week, and Dr S is helping her to prepare for it. Dr S is rather annoyed that these days there are annual fees for medical school. It's not really fair. Education should be free and accessible to everyone.

Dr S may have a great deal of empathy for Sally's circumstances, but the economic, social and educational attainment gap between them is enormous. Of course it is not Dr S's fault that Sally is struggling with the burden of childcare and lack of qualifications. Nor can it possibly be a GP's responsibility that waiting lists for non-private patients are so long. However, health professionals, especially doctors who earn a good wage, need to be aware of the image that they portray to their patients. High incomes combined with moaning about rising costs, dilution of professional autonomy and the necessity to prove competence will not improve the profession's image with the general public.

The scenario involving Dr S and Sally M also illustrates the gap in lifestyle and experience that lies between many doctors and their patients. Not only do we need to explore and develop sensitivity to cultural diversity, but also we should apply the same principles to social diversity. In simple terms, health professionals need to listen to the patient's voice, through education, talking to people, working in and engaging with diverse communities, and studying the humanities, as discussed in Chapter 10.

ALTRUISM

BOX 12.5 A DEFINITION OF ALTRUISM

Disinterested and selfless concern for the well-being of others; the performance of cooperative, unselfish acts that are beneficial to others.

Speaking out about social injustice and healthcare inequity may be seen as an example of altruistic behaviour, as may providing free healthcare when one is legally able to charge. In an editorial in the *British Medical Journal*, Roger Jones (a professor of general practice in the UK) wrote about the apparent decline in altruism in doctors. He cites as one example of this the decline in home-visiting rates by GPs[11] (an example that shows how differently altruism may be defined). Another example would be the reluctance of many doctors to provide a 24-hour service to patients. Altruism is dying at the expense of self-care – two aspects of professionalism pulling in opposite directions. Professor Jones suggests that cooperative behaviour towards another is more likely to occur when there is a direct or indirect benefit to be gained from altruistic behaviour (which rather goes against the definition). Such benefits include the esteem in which doctors are held and the level of remuneration that they receive for their services.[11] As noted in previous chapters, such esteem is being eroded, while many doctors feel that they are underpaid for the work they do.

IMPROVING HEALTH: A SOCIAL JUSTICE FRAMEWORK

The Scottish Executive in its Social Justice Annual Report at the turn of the twentieth century defined a number of conditions necessary to improve the health and social well-being of the population of Scotland.[12] Conditions directly relating to the work of health professionals are listed in Box 12.6. This list gives an indication of professional responsibility in relation to counselling and health promotion. We could say that in order to meet these challenges, a decent public health and education policy is needed, and that this is a political responsibility. Of course this is true, but individual health professionals are able to influence patients slowly over time, through empathy, communication and role modelling.

BOX 12.6 SOCIAL JUSTICE FOR SCOTLAND[12]

- Improving the well-being of young children by reducing the proportion of women who smoke during pregnancy, by reducing the percentage of low-birth-weight babies, and by increasing the number of women who breastfeed.
- Reducing smoking by 12- to 15-year-olds, teenage pregnancies, and the rate of suicide among young people.
- Improving the health of people by reducing smoking, alcohol abuse, poor diet and mortality rates from ischaemic heart disease.
- Increasing the number of old people who take regular physical exercise.
- Reducing the incidence of drug misuse in general, and of injections and needle sharing in particular.

RATIONING AND SOCIAL JUSTICE

The British National Health Service was established by the then Labour Government in 1948 to provide healthcare to the population on the basis of universality, comprehensiveness and free access.[13] Treatment was to be given to patients on the basis of need rather than their ability or willingness to pay. There was to be no discrimination with regard to gender, age, ethnic background, social class or religion. Healthcare would be of equal quality wherever it was delivered in the country. Every type of treatment would be available.

The aspirations of the founding fathers are well known. The NHS would be so successful in improving the health of the nation that eventually the service would be rarely needed. Of course in reality costs kept on rising, and they continue to do so as people live longer, medicine advances and new treatment modalities appear. Now the big debate is this. What is a patient's need? Moreover, who is to decide?

The definitions of need are debated by ethicists, philosophers, economists, politicians and health professionals. There is no one satisfactory answer. A doctor may advocate an individual patient's needs, or may take a public and population health perspective and look at decisions based on improving the lot of every citizen. If, as has been argued by some doctors, health professionals were not to consider costs when treating individual patients,[14] resources would soon be consumed, leading to worse inequity, as in time only those who were able to pay would be able to be treated. In professional practice we grapple with such decisions every day. Which drug should be prescribed? (Cost versus effectiveness versus evidence versus patient preference versus side-effect profile versus personal experience versus 'What would I want my mother to have?'). Does this patient need to be investigated? The patient expects an X-ray, but is this necessary apart from providing reassurance to the patient? Many of the decisions are made for health professionals by lack of availability, waiting lists and budgets. Although health professionals cannot avoid being involved in making resource decisions at an individual level, they are poorly qualified and usually untrained to do so, and often there are major conflicts of interest.[15]

Rather than consider the principles underlying rationing decisions, the philosophers Daniels and Sabin have suggested four conditions for setting limits to increase legitimacy and promote fairness (*see* Box 12.7).[16] (The word 'rationing' may be substituted for limit setting in this context.)

BOX 12.7 CONDITIONS FOR SETTING LIMITS[16]

Publicity condition: Decisions about the introduction of new technologies and their rationale must be publicly accessible.

Relevance condition: The rationale for limit-setting decisions should aim to provide a reasonable explanation of how the organisation (or society) should provide 'value for money' in meeting the varied health needs of a defined population under reasonable resource constraints.

Appeals condition: There should be a mechanism for challenge and resolution of disputes with regard to limit-setting decisions, including the opportunity to revise decisions in the light of further evidence or arguments.

Enforcement condition: There is either voluntary or public regulation of the process to ensure that the first three conditions are met.

Roger Crisp, a philosopher at Oxford University, has analysed to what extent the NHS still ensures that patients are treated according to need. He believes that a fundamental problem is that no one has ever defined what exactly in the way of healthcare the NHS should be delivering. Some hospital trusts have listed what they will not deliver (usually such procedures as tattoo removal and breast augmentation), but even the *NHS Plan* of 2000 does not tackle the issue of what should be rationed. Indeed the Plan states that 'The NHS will provide a comprehensive range of services.'[17]

A similar problem relates back to the proposal that there is a natural right to healthcare. The quote from the World Health Organization at the beginning of the chapter refers to the 'highest attainable standard of health', not a right to healthcare, although it may be assumed that the latter is necessary for the former. But what is healthcare?

Other countries are grappling with similar problems. The publicity relating to healthcare rationing is usually reported with an emphasis on cost. Governments know that promising extra money for healthcare is a vote winner, although extra money in itself will not solve the issues relating to spiralling healthcare costs. There will never be enough money to provide a universal, comprehensive health service, free at the point of delivery.

What is the professional viewpoint about inequity of service delivery? In countries where public and private healthcare is available, many doctors and health professionals work in both sectors. Patients who are told that they will have to wait 6 months to see Dr X at the public hospital might wonder at Dr X's free appointment next week at the private facility. Although poorer patients in the richer countries of the world have equal (and sometimes better) access to primary care and GPs, they have worse access to specialist care, particularly in those countries in which healthcare is partially funded by private insurance.[18]

Another American philosopher takes a hard line on rights even against his peers: 'Philosophers have acted no better than populist lobbyists in elevating the notion of a right to healthcare to the status of objective fact. There is no such right in general and, in particular, it is to be found only within the confines of a few medically enlightened nations. Even here it is a niggardly thing, graced with fine words but in practice an impoverished provision. I believe that the competition to expand health services to meet healthcare expectations will be the main social battlefield of the 21st century. As life's horizon extends for some, all others will feel cheated for being left behind, and left behind by their own national guardians.'[19]

DECIDING ON THE IMPLEMENTATION OF NEW TREATMENTS

Although many rationing decisions affect treatments that are already tried and tested and have some form of evidence base, consensus needs to be reached on whether new, and in all likelihood expensive, therapies should be introduced. Or rather whether such treatments should be available within a state- or insurance-funded system, as they may well be deemed suitable for private fee-paying patients. In the UK, such decisions are made by health authorities. In other countries they are made by health insurers. In most cases cost-effectiveness is taken into account.

The quality-adjusted life year (QALY) is such a measure of cost-effectiveness. One QALY is one year of healthy life expectancy, whereas a year of unhealthy life expectancy is worth less than one. The quality of the unhealthy life determines the value.[20]

Hope and colleagues from the University of Oxford have devised a four-step model to help budget allocation bodies to decide whether to fund a new treatment (*see* Box 12.8).[21] This method seeks to answer questions about whether there is satisfactory evidence, and how reliable it is, whether the treatment is effective and whether it is worth paying the cost, given the value of the effect. Moreover, the answers to these questions are also dependent on the money that the service has available. The costs of some interventions are just too expensive, regardless of their effectiveness. Such a transparent method should allow health professionals to justify to their patients why certain advertised treatments are not available. What we could say in such circumstances is therefore a more professional approach to healthcare rationing. After all, it is usually a health professional, not a politician or budget negotiator, who has to deal with individual patients requesting new interventions.

BOX 12.8 A FOUR-STEP METHOD FOR DECIDING
WHETHER TO FUND NEW TREATMENTS

- Collect evidence with regard to how much the treatment costs per life year extended (or QALY).
- Compare this cost with how much money the funding body has available per QALY.
- If the proposed treatment falls within the budget, assume that the treatment should be provided.
- If the proposed treatment costs more, decide whether there are grounds for paying more than the usual amount per QALY, and whether the extra money is justified.

There are of course ethical issues relating to all such decisions. Are the decisions fair or discriminatory? Although a majority opinion working within a social justice framework would state that it is unfair to ration on the basis of a patient's gender or race, some analysts feel that decisions based on age are only logical. After all, everyone ages, so there is the potential for all of us to be submitted to rationing, but we cannot change our ethnic origin (nor in most circumstances our gender).[8]

Rationing impinges on a professional's sense of fairness. Altruism is seen as a hallmark of professionalism. Rationing offends the sense of selfless concern. On the whole, professionals want what is best for their patients. When rationing is imposed, there is the rationale to accept what cannot be changed and to inform patients of this. However, some will speak out against what they see as inequity within the system.

SUMMARY

In this book we have offered various perspectives on professionalism, dissecting the concept into various components while providing both an evidence-based and personal approach. The literature on professionalism is growing exponentially. The big issues include teaching and learning professionalism, the assessment of professional behaviour at all levels of practice, and the problem of what should happen when professionals are deemed to be acting 'unprofessionally.' Professionalism also encompasses self-care, lifelong learning, teamwork and interaction within a culturally diverse society.

Health professionals will increasingly be faced with ethical decisions relating to rationing, quality of life, euthanasia and assisted suicide, and the sequelae of the widening gap between rich and poor, both within and between nations. Some will feel that they should champion their patients' needs on a wider scale than the individual patient–professional relationship. Such battles have implications for their own health and priorities with regard to work and family.

There are as many questions as there are answers, and many opinions and areas of research. However, we hope that our thoughts and writing have contributed to the discussion and exploration of this important topic.

REFERENCES

1 www.who.int/about/definition/en/ (accessed July 2005).
2 Medical Professionalism Project; www.acponline.org/journals/news/jul01/professionalism.htm (accessed May 2008).
3 Smith R. The failings of NICE. *BMJ.* 2000; **321**: 1363–4.
4 Soanes C, Stevenson A, editors. *Oxford Dictionary of English.* 2nd ed. Oxford: Oxford University Press; 2003.
5 www.unhchr.ch/udhr/index.htm (accessed May 2008).
6 Department of Health and Social Security. *Inequalities in Health: report of a research working group (Black Report).* London: Department of Health and Social Security; 1980.
7 Smith JD. *Australia's Rural and Remote Health. A social justice perspective.* Victoria: Tertiary Press; 2004.
8 Daniels N. Justice, health and health care. In: Rhodes R, Battin MP, Silvers A, editors. *Medicine and Social Justice. Essays on the distribution of health care.* Oxford: Oxford University Press; 2002. pp. 6–23.
9 Wilkinson RG. *Unhealthy Societies: the afflictions of inequality.* London: Routledge; 1996.
10 Couzos S, Murray R, editors. *Aboriginal Primary Health Care. An evidence-based approach.* 2nd ed. Melbourne: Oxford University Press; 2003.
11 Jones R. Declining altruism in medicine. *BMJ.* 2002; **324**: 624–5.
12 www.scotland.gov.uk/library5/social/emsjm-00.asp (accessed May 2008).
13 Webster C. *The National Health Service.* Oxford: Oxford University Press; 1998.
14 Abrams F. The doctor with two heads – the patient versus the costs. *NEJM.* 1994; **328**: 975–7.
15 Kerridge I, Lowe M, McPhee J. *Ethics and Law for the Health Professions.* 2nd ed. Sydney: The Federation Press; 2005.
16 Daniels N, Sabin J. Limits to health care: fair procedures, democratic deliberation, and the legitimacy problem for insurers. *Philos Public Affairs.* 1997; **26**: 303–50.
17 Department of Health. *The NHS Plan: a plan for investment, a plan for reform.* London: Department of Health; 2000.

18 Baumrin BH. Why there is no right to health care. In: Rhodes R, Battin MP, Silvers A, editors. *Medicine and Social Justice. Essays on the distribution of health care.* Oxford: Oxford University Press; 2002. pp. 78–83.

19 Spurgeon D. Poor patients in rich countries have fair access to GPs but not to specialists. *BMJ.* 2006; **332**: 138.

20 Williams A. QALYs and ethics – a health economist's view. *Soc Sci Med.* 1996; **43**: 1795–804.

21 Hope T, Reynolds J, Griffiths S. Rationing decisions: integrating cost-effectiveness with other values. In: Rhodes R, Battin MP, Silvers A, editors. *Medicine and Social Justice. Essays on the distribution of health care.* Oxford: Oxford University Press; 2002. pp. 144–55.

Index

abbreviations 74
Aborigines 213
abortion 37, 38, 41, 42
accountability 10, 12, 153
acronyms 74
Aesculapian power 59
affective processes 162–4
Agate, James 1
aggressive patients 58
alcoholism 118, 119, 120, 127, 131, 144
Alder Hey Hospital 140, 150
altruism 7, 12, 14, 65, 215–16, 220
American Board of Internal Medicine (ABIM) 6, 210
American College of Physicians 6, 210
angry patients 58
anxiety 119, 122
apothecaries 22, 23
appraisal 4, 127, 141, 142, 180, 196
Aristotle 104
Arnold, L 190
arts 174–7
Ashworth Hospital 140
Askham, Janet 13
assault 48, 57
assessing professionalism 185–209
    assessment by peers 202–5
    communication 199–202
    learning and teaching professionalism 166, 180
    literature review 190–2
    overview 185–6
    portfolio-based assessment 196–9
    reflection and self-assessment 195–6
    requirements for assessment 189–90
    responding to lapses 205–6
    summary 206–7
    utility of assessment 187–9
    why assess? 186–7
    workplace-based assessment 192–5
assisted suicide 42, 221

attitudes 79–80
audit 145–7
Australia 94, 124, 213–14
autonomy
    code of conduct, law and ethics 42, 43
    ethics and the law 170
    evolution of the professions 18–19
    informed choice and informed consent 80
    nature of autonomy 134–55
        clinical autonomy and clinical audit 145–7
        complaints against doctors 144–5
        de-professionalisation 148–50
        GMC and self-regulation 137–9
        GMC in the twenty-first century 142–3
        GMC up to 2008 141
        maintaining professionalism 152
        overview 134–5
        patient autonomy and rise of consumerism 150–2
        professional autonomy 135–7
        revalidation 141–2
        role of public inquiries 140
        whistleblowing 143–4
    North American developments 7
    patient-centred professionalism 14

battery 48, 81
Beauchamp, TL 43
Bentham, Jeremy 40
Berns, Kenneth 9
best-evidence medical education (BEME) 178
Bevan, Aneurin 26
Beveridge Report (1942) 26
Black Report 212
Blair, Tony 29
'Blue Book' 4
BMA Counselling Service 131
Bolam v Friern Hospital Management Committee 48
Bolitho v City and Hackney HA 49

Bolsin, Steve 143
boundary violations 60–2
Bristol Inquiry (1998) 5–6, 77, 138–9, 140, 150, 169
British Medical Association (BMA)
    communication 75
    learning from history 26, 30
    personal development and self-care 119, 123, 129
    physical and sexual harassment 57
    recent interest in professionalism 3
British Medical Journal 30, 42, 122, 128, 215
Brody, H 52, 59
Browne-Wilkinson, Lord 49
burnout 122–3, 127, 128, 176

Calgary–Cambridge framework 169–70, 199
Calman, Sir Kenneth 3
CanMEDS 9, 161, 196
Carr-Saunders, AM 29
categorical imperative 40
Catto, Graeme 139
Cayton, Harry 14
CBD (case-based discussion) 195
Centre for the Advancement of Interprofessional Education (CAIPE) 84
Chambers, R 111
chaperones 56–7
charismatic power 59
Charles, C 80–1
Childress, J 43
Chisholm, Alison 13
Clance Scale 121
clinical audit 145–7
clinical autonomy 145–7, 148, 149
clinical governance 141, 146, 147, 159
clinical quality 146–7
Cochrane Collaboration 114
code of conduct 36–51
    deciding on an ethical code 43–4
    duties of a doctor 40–2
    ethical, legal and professional duties 38–9
    ethics in medicine 39–40
    first, do no harm 46–7
    Good Samaritan 46
    medical malpractice 48–9
    overview 36–7
    patient safety 47
    patients' rights 44–5
    professional versus private code of conduct 37–8
    summary 49
    where to find help 49
cognitive processes 162–4
Commission for Health Improvement (CHI) 140
communication 69–88
    art of communication 70–2
    assessing professionalism 199–202

autonomy 144, 150
barriers to good communication 75–6
behaviour and attitudes 79–80
communicating with patients and the public 77–9
confidentiality 85–6
cultural diversity 98
dysfunctional teams 83–4
informed choice and informed consent 80–1
interprofessional communication and teams 82–3
interprofessional education 84–5
is there a problem? 72–3
learning and teaching professionalism 159, 167–70
miscommunication 73–5
outcomes of poor communication 76–7
overview 69–70
communication skills teaching (CST) 169
compensation 38, 144, 145
competence 107, 189, 192, 193, 200
complaints 47, 119, 127, 144–5, 150
complementary medicine 22, 24, 25
confidentiality 40, 54, 76, 85–6, 97
consent 46, 48, 80–1, 85, 86, 201
consequentialism 39, 40
consequential validity 189
construct validity 188
consumerism 150–2
content validity 188–9
continuing medical education (CME) 105
continuing professional development (CPD) 105–7, 141, 142, 157, 178, 180
continuing professional education (CPE) 107
cost-effectiveness 219
Coull, R 143
Coulter, Angela 77
counselling services 131
counter-transference 60, 61
creative writing 174–7
Crisp, Roger 218
criterion validity 189
Cruess, Richard 9, 30, 31, 158, 159
Cruess, Sylvia 9, 30, 31, 158, 159
cultural diversity 89–101
    culture of medical profession 93
    culture shock 99
    definitions 90–1
    diversity wheel 92–3
    exploring health beliefs 95–7
    learning and teaching professionalism 159
    multicultural health service 97
    overview 89–90
    professional approach to racism 98–9
    reflections on teaching cultural diversity 93–5
    social justice 213–14
culture 91, 92, 93
culture shock 99

Daniels, Norman 212, 217
death 128
defensive strategies 65, 66
deontology 41
Department of Health 47, 48, 117, 119, 126, 142
depression 119, 122
de-professionalisation 148–50
Developing Medical Regulation (GMC) 139
Diagnostic and Statistical Manual of Mental Disorders (DSM-IV) 96
DIPEX (Database of Personal Experience of Health and Illness) 177
direct observation 200, 201
disease–illness framework 169
distribution of wealth 212
diversity wheel 92–3
doctors
    autonomy 144–5
    context of professionalism 1–2, 3
    duties of a doctor 4, 40–2, 45, 46
    elements of a profession 18
    personal development and self-care
        acting as a doctor's doctor 129–30
        causes of ill health 120–1
        doctors' health-seeking behaviour 123–6
        maintaining one's health 118–19
    social justice 214–15
A Doctor's Dilemma (Shaw) 2
Doctors' Support Network 131
The Doctors' Tale (Irvine) 137
Donabedian, A 146, 147
Donaldson, Liam 117, 180
DOPS (direct observation of procedural skills) 195
drug abuse 119, 120, 127, 131, 144, 206
drug industry 63–4, 172
duties of a doctor 4, 40–2, 45, 46, 48, 49
Duties of a Doctor (GMC) 4
duty of care 48, 49

Edelstein, Ludwig 20
education
    autonomy 142, 143
    cultural diversity 93–5
    interprofessional education 84–5
    learning and teaching professionalism
        communication 167–70
        context 158
        ethics and the law 170–3
        fostering self-awareness 173–4
        framework for development 162–4
        hidden curriculum 166–7
        interprofessional education and learning 178
        involving patients 177–8
        learner's perspective 180–1
        learning environment 166
        outcome-based approach 164–5

        patient safety 178–80
        PDPs, appraisal and revalidation 180
        role of humanities 174–7
        some educational considerations 161–2
    personal development and self-care 127–8
educational climate 166
educational needs assessment 108–10
Einstein, Albert 165
Eisenberg, John 162
embedded approach 170, 171, 172
empathy 64–6, 128–9, 177, 200
empirical empathy 129
end-of-life decisions 172
epilepsy 39
Epstein, RE 191
Eraut, Michael 69, 103, 104, 106, 107
errors
    autonomy 140, 150
    communication 77
    learning and teaching professionalism 173, 178–80
    patient safety 47
    personal development and self-care 119, 127
Escott, THS 17
ethics
    code of conduct, law and ethics
        deciding on an ethical code 43–4
        ethical, legal and professional duties 38–9
        ethics in medicine 39–40
        overview 36, 37
        professional versus private code of conduct 37–8
        where to find help 49
    communication 86, 201
    learning and teaching professionalism 159, 170–3
    personal development and self-care 123–4
    social justice 210, 211, 220, 221
ethnicity 92, 93, 95
European Federation of Internal Medicine 6, 210
European Working Time Directive 121
euthanasia 37, 221
Evans, R 202
evidence-based medicine (EBM) 111–13
evidence of learning 110–11
expert patients 177

face validity 188
family members 55, 86
female genital mutilation 97
fitness to practise 141, 142, 170, 205
Flexner, Abraham 156
formative assessment 188, 201
Foucault, Michel 135
Foundation Programme 4, 159, 202
free market 151

Freidson, Eliot
  autonomy 135, 145, 150, 151, 152
  communication 73
  learning from history 17, 18, 19, 29
  medical power 59
fundholding 28, 137, 148

Gabbay, J 113
General Medical Council (GMC)
  assessing professionalism 196, 205
  autonomy 137–9, 141, 142–3, 144
  code of conduct, law and ethics 36, 37, 38,
    42, 46
  communication 79–80, 85
  cultural diversity 94
  learning and teaching professionalism
    159
  learning from history 23–6, 30, 32
  patient-centred professionalism 14
  personal development and self-care 123,
    131
  professional–patient relationships 54, 55,
    62
  recent interest in professionalism 3, 4, 5, 6
General Practice Assessment Questionnaire
  (GPAQ) 201
General Practice Assessment Survey (GPAS)
  201
Gerstl, J 19
gifts 62–3, 63–4
Ginsburg, S 191
global rating scales 194
GMC *see* General Medical Council
The Good CPD Guide 109
Good Doctors, Safer Patients 142, 180
Good Medical Practice (GMC) 4, 5, 14, 37,
  79–80, 159, 160–1
Good Samaritan 46
Gordon, Jill 162, 164, 180
governmentality 135
GP contract 137, 146, 150, 201
Grant, Janet 109

Hafferty, Fred 207
Hall, Katherine 55
Hamilton, John 165
harassment 57–8
Harvey Scale 121
Hayek, Friedrich 27
health
  causes of ill health 120–1
  doctors' health-seeking behaviour 123–6
  maintaining one's health 118–19
  recognising problems in oneself and others
    130–1
  social justice 210–11, 212, 213, 218
Health Act (1999) 29
health beliefs 95–7
health services market models 151–2
Henry VIII 21

hidden curriculum 104, 157, 166, 166–7, 180,
  181
Higgins, J 140
Higson, R 175
Hilton, SR 2, 9–10, 180
Hippocrates 20, 46
Hippocratic Oath 20–1, 36, 53
HIV (human immunodeficiency virus) 39, 40,
  172
home visits 149, 216
Hope, T 219
humanities 174–7
humour 128, 167
Hundert, EM 191
hypochondriasis 128, 130

Illich, Ivan 2, 27, 28
illness framework 169
illness scripts 113
Imes, SA 121
immunisation 39–40, 150
imposter syndrome 121–2
Improving Working Lives Standard 126
incognito standardised patients (ISPs) 201
indigenous nations 213, 214
industrialisation of medicine 6, 8
information overload 113–14
informed choice 80–1
informed consent 46, 80–1
institutional racism 98
institutional slang 167
internal market 27–8
internal reliability 189
International Covenant on Economic, Social
  and Cultural Rights 44, 45
Internet 69, 70
interpreters 76, 96
interprofessional communication 82–3
interprofessional education (IPE) 84–5,
  178
intimate examinations 48, 53, 54, 55, 56–7
Irvine, Sir Donald 5, 137, 138, 139
Irvine, R 94

Jacobs, G 19
jargon 73, 74, 76
Jewell, David 141
John Paul II, Pope 85
Johnson, T 136
Jones, Roger 215–16
Journal of Medical Ethics 175
just (definition) 211
justice (definition) 211

Kant, Immanuel 40
Kennedy, Professor Ian 5
Kennedy Report 5, 6, 10
Kerridge, Ian 43, 54
King's Fund 11
Kirkpatrick, DI 84

Klein, R 30
knowledge 103–4

Lancet 6
language barriers 70, 75–6, 96, 98
Larkin, G 26
Larson, MS 24–5
Latin language 23, 73, 74
law 36–51
    deciding on an ethical code 43–4
    duties of a doctor 40–2
    ethical, legal and professional duties 38–9
    ethics in medicine 39–40
    first, do no harm 46–7
    Good Samaritan 46
    learning and teaching professionalism 170–3
    medical malpractice 48–9
    overview 36–7
    patient safety 47
    patients' rights 44–5
    professional versus private code of conduct 37–8
    where to find help 49
Lawrence, Stephen 89, 98
Leape, Lucian 178
Learning and Teaching Support Network (LTSN) 85
learning environment 166
learning needs 108–10
learning outcomes 164–5
Ledward, Rodney 5, 140
Leicester Assessment Package 201
Leininger, MM 97
le May, A 113
Levinson, Wendy 77
Libertarian Alliance 30
life expectancy 212, 213, 219
lifelong learning 102, 103, 195
Light, Donald 136, 137, 148
Lynch, DC 190

Macpherson Report 98
malpractice 48–9
Mandell, HN 128
media 70, 85, 150, 206
Medical Acts 24, 25, 137
Medical Council of New Zealand 55, 56
medical education *see* education
Medical Education 121, 175
medical errors *see* errors
medical humanities 174–7
medical malpractice 48–9
medical power 58–60
Medical Professionalism Project 6, 102, 210
Medical Schools Council (MSC) 14
medical students 125, 126, 127, 129, 158, 180
Medical Students: Professional Behaviour and Fitness to Practise (MSC) 14

mental health
    assessing professionalism 206
    complaints 144
    cultural diversity 96
    personal development and self-care 119, 125, 127, 128
Mental Health Act 42
mentoring 127
meta-analyses 114
metacognitive processes 162–4
Miller's pyramid 192, 193
mini-CEX (mini-clinical evaluation exercise) 195, 200
miniPAT (peer assessment tool) 202, 203–4, 205
miscommunication 73–5
misconduct 38, 54, 55, 62, 142
moral law 40
morbidity data 119, 212, 213
Morris, P 199
mortality data 119, 212, 213
multiculturalism 89, 90, 97
multi-source feedback (MSF) 202

narrative approaches 174–7
National Clinical Assessment Authority (NCAA) 140
National Counselling Service for Sick Doctors (NCSSD) 131
National Health Service and Community Care Act (1990) 28
National Health Service Executive 77
National Health Service (NHS)
    autonomy 137, 140, 143, 144, 145
    communication 72, 73, 74
    learning from history 26–9, 32, 33–4
    patient safety 47
    personal development and self-care 126
    social justice 217, 218
National Institute for Clinical Excellence (NICE) 146
National Institute for Health and Clinical Excellence (NICE) 95, 211
National Patient Safety Agency (NPSA) 78, 140, 180
natural empathy 129
Neale, Richard 5
needs assessment 108–10
negligence 38, 48, 49, 81, 144, 145, 173
The New NHS 146
NHS Litigation Authority 144
The NHS Plan 137, 150, 218
Norcini, John 195
Nuffield Trust 120

Objective Structured Clinical Examination (OSCE) 188, 199–200
O'Neill, Onora 10–11
An Organisation with a Memory (DoH) 47
Osler, Sir William 117, 177
outcome-based approach 164–5

Parsons, Talcot 27, 30, 31, 141
paternalism 30, 31, 58, 73, 78, 96, 152
patient autonomy 150–2
patient-centred professionalism 13–14, 58, 95, 96
patient partnership 77, 78, 79, 151, 177–8
patient safety 47, 159, 178–80
Patient's Charter 59, 151
peer assessment 202–5
Percival, Thomas 31
performance 107, 189, 192, 193, 200, 205, 206
personal development
    learning and teaching professionalism 162–4
    personal development and self-care 117–33
        acting as a doctor's doctor 129–30
        causes of ill health 120–1
        doctors' health-seeking behaviour 123–6
        education and prevention 127–8
        imposter syndrome 121–2
        initiatives to improve well-being 126–7
        learning from others' stories 128–9
        maintaining one's health 118–19
        overview 117–18
        recognising problems 130–1
        sick doctors 119–20
        unhappy or burnt out? 122–3
personal development plans (PDPs) 107–10, 141, 180
pharmaceutical companies 63–4, 172
PHOG (Prejudice, Hunch, Opinion, Guesswork) 187
physical harassment 57–8
Picker Institute Europe 72, 73
Popper, Karl 36
Porter, Roy 22
portfolios 107–8, 180, 196–9
postcode rationing 33
Postgraduate Medical Education and Training Board 143
power 58–60
Powley, E 175
practical knowledge 104
practice-based commissioning (PBC) 137
pragmatic approach 170
predictive validity 189
prejudice 90, 98
Prescription Medicine Code of Practice Authority 64
Primary Care Assessment Survey 201
primary care trusts (PCTs) 29
Pringle, Mike 141
Private Eye 5
Private Finance Initiative (PFI) 29
private patients 151
professional autonomy 134, 135–7
professional development 158, 162–4, 180
professionalism
    assessing professionalism 185–209

    assessment by peers 202–5
    communication 199–202
    literature review 190–2
    overview 185–6
    portfolio-based assessment 196–9
    reflection and self-assessment 195–6
    requirements for assessment 189–90
    responding to lapses 205–6
    summary 206–7
    utility of assessment 187–9
    why assess? 186–7
    workplace-based assessment 192–5
autonomy 152
code of conduct, law and ethics 36–51
    deciding on an ethical code 43–4
    duties of a doctor 40–2
    ethical, legal and professional duties 38–9
    ethics in medicine 39–40
    first, do no harm 46–7
    Good Samaritan 46
    medical malpractice 48–9
    overview 36–7
    patient safety 47
    patients' rights 44–5
    professional versus private code of conduct 37–8
    summary 49
    where to find help 49
communication 69–88
    art of communication 70–2
    barriers to good communication 75–6
    behaviour and attitudes 79–80
    communicating with patients and the public 77–9
    confidentiality 85–6
    dysfunctional teams 83–4
    informed choice and informed consent 80–1
    interprofessional communication and teams 82–3
    interprofessional education 84–5
    is there a problem? 72–3
    miscommunication 73–5
    outcomes of poor communication 76–7
    overview 69–70
context 1–16
    definitions of professionalism 2
    developments in North America 6–9
    historical context 1–2
    origins of recent interest 3–6
    patient-centred professionalism 13–14
    professionalism must be taught 9–10
    a question of trust 10–13
culture of medical profession 93
learning and teaching professionalism 156–84
    communication 167–70
    context 157–61

ethics and the law 170–3
fostering self-awareness 173–4
framework for development 162–4
hidden curriculum 166–7
interprofessional education and learning 178
involving patients 177–8
learner's perspective 180–1
learning environment 166
outcome-based approach 164–5
overview 156
patient safety 178–80
PDPs, appraisal and revalidation 180
some educational considerations 161–2
summary 181–2
learning from history 17–35
American experience 33
control and certification 21–3
elements of a profession 17–18
evolution of the professions 18–20
the healer versus the professional 30–3
Hippocrates and the Greek tradition 20–1
internal market 27–8
National Health Service 26–7
National Health Service under New Labour 29
professionalisation of medicine 24–6
summary 33–4
writing about the professions 29–30
social justice 210–22
altruism 215–16
definitions 211–13
doctors' place in society 214–15
example from Australia 213–14
improving health: a social justice framework 216
new treatments 219–20
overview 210–11
rationing healthcare 217–19
summary 220–1
professional knowledge and development 102–16
Cochrane Collaboration 114
competence and performance 107
continuing professional development 105–7
evidence-based medicine 111–12
evidence of learning 110–11
information overload 113–14
nature of professional knowledge 103–4
overview 102–3
personal development plans 107–10
problems with evidence-based approach 111–12
work-based learning and reflection 114
youth versus experience 104–5
professional–patient relationships 52–68
boundary violations 60–2
chaperones and intimate examinations 56–7
doctor–patient sexual relationships 53–5
drug industry 63–4
empathy 64–6
former patients 55–6
medical power 58–60
overview 52–3
physical and sexual harassment by patients 57–8
receiving gifts 62–3
propositional knowledge 104
proto-professionalism 180
pseudo-empathy 65
pseudo-teams 83
psychiatrists 54, 55
Public Disclosure Act 143
public inquiries 140

qualitative reviews 114
quality-adjusted life year (QALY) 219, 220
quality of care 146–7

race 92–3, 95
racism 42, 76, 79, 89, 90, 98–9
rationing healthcare 211, 217–21
recertification 142
reflection 161, 195–6
regulation 139, 142
reliability 187, 188, 189, 195, 198
relicensure 142
religion 41
remediation 205–6
retirement 105
revalidation 4, 105, 108, 141–2, 143, 180
Revill, J 143
rights
    autonomy 151
    code of conduct, law and ethics 40, 41, 44–5
    social justice 210, 211, 218, 219
    trust 10
Roskam, John 89
Royal College of General Practitioners (RCGP) 200
Royal College of Obstetricians and Gynaecologists 48, 56–7
Royal College of Physicians and Surgeons (Canada) 8–9, 161
Royal College of Physicians 11, 12, 23, 64
Royal College of Surgeons 23
Royal Colleges 105, 141, 142
Rughani, A 108

Sabin, J 217
Sackin, Paul 65
safety *see* patient safety
Salinsky, John 65
Scarman, Lord 49
Schofield, T 168

Schön, DA 103–4
Scottish Executive 216
sectioning patients 42
self-assessment 195–6
self-awareness 173–4, 177
self-care
    personal development and self-care 117–33
        acting as a doctor's doctor 129–30
        causes of ill health 120–1
        doctors' health-seeking behaviour
            123–6
        education and prevention 127–8
        imposter syndrome 121–2
        initiatives to improve well-being 126–7
        learning from others' stories 128–9
        maintaining one's health 118–19
        overview 117–18
        recognising problems 130–1
        sick doctors 119–20
        unhappy or burnt out? 122–3
    social justice 216
self-medication 125
self-regulation 137–9
sexual relationships 52–8, 60–2
Shaw, George Bernard 2
Sheffield Peer Review Assessment Tool
    (SPRAT) 202, 205
Shipman, Harold 5, 6, 127, 139–41, 150
Shock, Sir Maurice 3–4, 5
sick leave 124
sickness in doctors
    acting as a doctor's doctor 129–30
    causes of ill health 120–1
    learning from others' stories 128–9
    maintaining one's health 118–19
    overview 117–18
    recognising problems 130–1
    sick doctors 119–20
Sidaway v Governors of Bethlem Royal Hospital 49
Slotnik, HB 2, 9–10, 180
SMART outcomes (Specific, Measurable,
    Achievable, Relevant, Timed) 165
Smith, Dame Janet 139, 141
Smith, Richard 5, 6, 122, 139, 146, 211
social justice 210–22
    altruism 215–16
    definitions 211–13
    doctors' place in society 214–15
    example from Australia 213–14
    improving health: a social justice
        framework 216
    new treatments 219–20
    North American developments 7
    overview 210–11
    rationing 217–19
    social justice – definitions 211

summary 220–1
social power 59
Spiro, Howard 64, 128
stability 189
Stacey, Meg 137
state 135, 136, 137, 148
Stephenson, A 157
Stern, David 191
stress 119, 121–3, 125, 127, 130
substance misuse 119, 120, 127, 131, 144, 206
suicide 119
summative assessment 188, 197, 198, 201
Swick, Herbert M 7–8
systematic reviews 114

*Taking Alcohol and Other Drugs out of the NHS
    Workplace* (DoH) 119
Tawney, RH 29
teamwork 82–4, 159, 178
technical knowledge 104
test–retest reliability 189
Thatcher, Margaret 27, 28
theoretical approach 170
Thistlethwaite, J 199
TLAs (three-letter acronyms) 74
Tolliday, H 145
Tomorrow's Doctors (GMC) 3, 159, 169
transcultural nursing movement 97
transference 60, 61
trust 10–13, 152
Trust, Assurance and Safety (GMC) 142

United Nations 44, 211
Universal Declaration of Human Rights 211
utilitarianism 40

validity 187, 188–9, 198
van der Vleuten, Cees 187, 189, 200
Veloski, JJ 190
videotaping consultations 200, 201
violence 57

waiting lists 28, 33
Walshe, K 140
Webb, Beatrice 29
Webb, Sidney 29
welfare state 27, 28
whistleblowing 143–4
work-based learning and reflection 114
Working for Patients 28, 146
working hours 120, 121
workplace-based assessment 192–5, 200
World Health Organization 146, 147, 210, 218
World Medical Association 134

Yeats, WB 5, 139